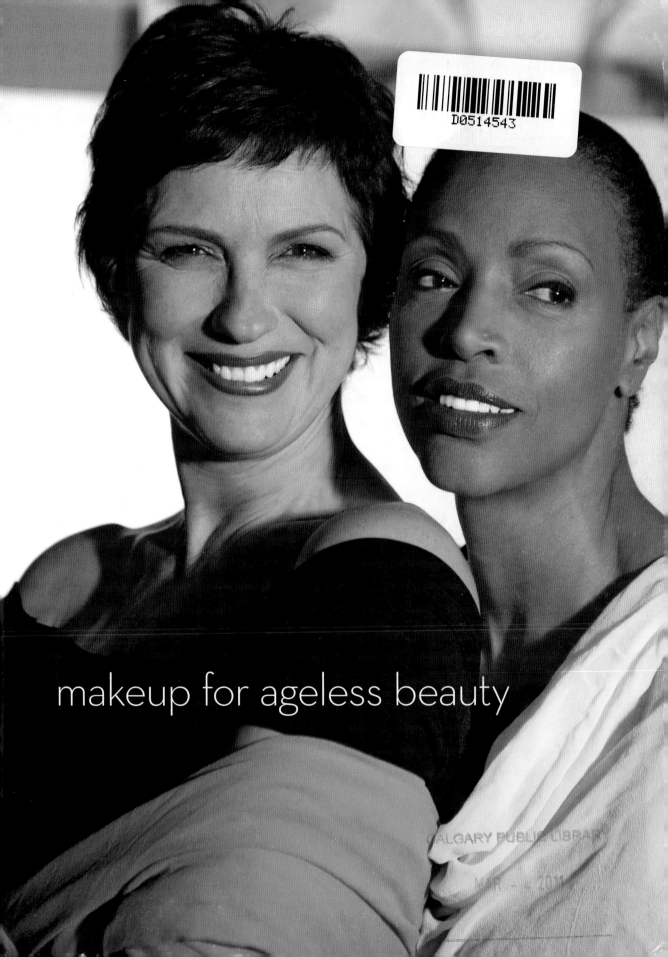

makeup for ageless beauty

D0514543

CALGARY PUBLIC LIBRARY

MAR - - 2011

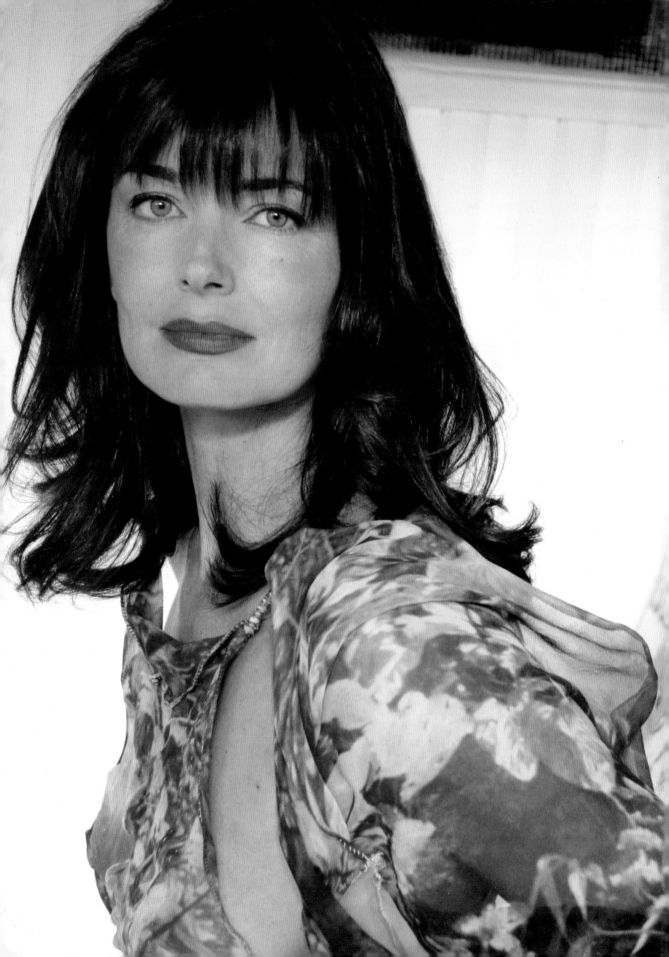

makeup for ageless beauty

MORE THAN 40 COLORFUL, CREATIVE LOOKS FOR WOMEN 40 AND OVER

linda mason

FOREWORD BY SHIRLEY LORD

WATSON-GUPTILL PUBLICATIONS / NEW YORK

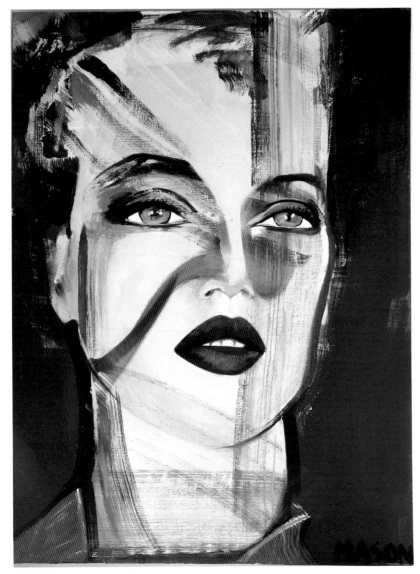

Marie Sophie by Linda Mason.

Copyright © 2011 by Linda Mason

All rights reserved.

First published in the United States in 2011 by Watson-Guptill Publications,
an imprint of the Crown Publishing Group,
a division of Random House, Inc.,
1745 Broadway, New York, NY 10019

WATSON-GUPTILL is a registered trademark and the WG and Horse designs are registered trademarks of Random House, Inc.

Library of Congress Cataloging-in-Publication Data

Mason, Linda.
  Makeup for ageless beauty : more than 40 colorful creative looks for women over 40 / Linda Mason ; foreword by Shirley Lord
      p. cm.
  ISBN-13: 978-0-8230-2479-7 (alk. paper)

  1. Cosmetics. 2. Middle-aged women—Health and hygiene. 3. Beauty, Personal. I. Title.
  RA778.M3765 2011
  613'.04244—dc22

2010036835

Printed in China

Cover and interior design by Marysarah Quinn
Cover and interior photos by Linda Mason except for page 10, center right, by Mario Arenas.

10 9 8 7 6 5 4 3 2 1

First Edition

acknowledgments

First and foremost, I'd like to thank my editor, Joy Aquilino, for entrusting me with this project, for her patience with me, and for doing such wonderful work clarifying my instructions. I'd also like to thank all the wonderful women from my past and present who have given so generously of their time to model for the book. It's been such a pleasure to catch up with them and once again to make up some of my favorite faces: Alva Chinn, Anna Bayle, Anne Bezamat, Barbara Nevins Taylor, Barbara Novogratz, Bibi Lencek, Brooke Shields, Carol Alt, Cécile Defforey, Christine De Lisle, Claudja Bicalho, Coco Mitchell, Dana Roc, Debbie Dickinson, Diana de Vegh, Doris Lozada, Felicia Milewicz, Finn O'Gorman, Frederique van der Wal, Grisel Baltazar, Gunilla Lindblad, Jan Jaffe, Joan Elizabeth Goodman, Joan Jett, Kikan Massara, Kim Alexis, Lilo Zinglersen, Margie Martin, Mimi Oka, Mimi Quillin, Silko Coelenbier, Nancy DeWeir Geaney, Paulina Porizkova, Phyllis Molle, Shirley Lord, Susanna Midnight, and Veronica Webb.

Thanks also go out to friends who have always been there to help me: Almog and Levi Okunov. Hairstylist Almog did the hair on Alva, Brooke, Carol, Doris, Debbie, Frederique, Gunilla, Kim, Kikan, Nancy, Paulina, Laura, Shirley, and Veronica; designer Levi lent the clothes for Brooke, Susanna, and Lilo to model. I would like to also thank hairstylist Tomoyasu Nakajima for his work on Joan Jett; Monica Castiglioni (www.monicacastiglioni.com) for the jewelry modeled by Carol Alt; Angela Garacija for the makeup on Phyllis; Kiara Vacchio for the makeup on Bibi; Venetia Stravens for the makeup on Mimi in the photo at the beginning of the book and Paula Quesada for makeup on Coco in the same photo. My agent, Jayne Rockmill, deserves thanks for her friendship and perseverance, as do developmental editor Amy Vinchesi for her great editing job and for doing wonders sorting through the material I gave her; art director Jess Morphew; creative director Marysarah Quinn; Meghan Hines for her research on cosmetic ingredients; and, last but not least, my interns Laura Buck and Elsa Bloedon.

contents

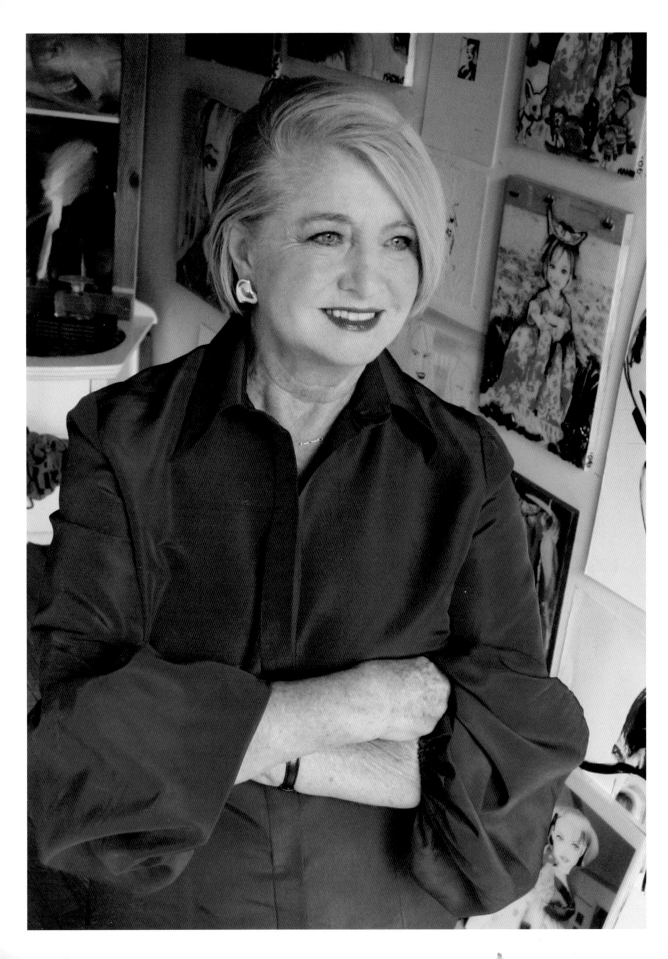

foreword Shirley Lord

Passersby on Grand Street in New York City tend to stop and stare at number 28, which is home to Linda Mason's makeup studio. Some are lured inside because the door is open and a magical, Wizard-of-Oz atmosphere beckons, an enticing view of makeup as transformation, as natural or as exotic as your persona desires and dictates.

Linda Mason, for some inexplicable reason, is not a household name, perhaps because, like selfish people everywhere, her aficionados rarely want to share her genius expertise, even with their nearest and dearest.

In this compelling book, Linda diffuses the magic behind the artifice and shows us in a clear, intelligent way how to make the most attractive versions of ourselves. Like a great chef, she picks the right ingredients and chooses the right tools to produce the finest results. For thirty-five years I have admired and respected Linda's use of color, brush, pen, pencil, and tweezer, creating younger out of older, extraordinary out of ordinary, and, above all, creating perfectly beautiful, believable makeup.

In the 1970s, as global vice president for Helena Rubinstein, I launched the first makeup made out of silk, in Como, the home of silk, on the shores of Lake Como in Italy. At the glamorous Villa D'Este, Linda was my right hand, and it was her amazing makeup that transformed the mature Veruschka's striking looks, which stunned the international press into awed silence as she entered the silk-lined ballroom (admittedly while sitting atop a white stallion).

I didn't think twice about asking Linda to accompany me on my tour of Britain to promote my book *You Are Beautiful and How to Prove It*. Her masterful skill helped me prove it on dozens and dozens of "before and after" volunteers, the majority well over 40.

As beauty director, first for *Harper's Bazaar* and then for *Vogue* (where I continue to serve as a contributing editor), I came to understand how makeup can truly be psychiatry for the face; not tyranny following "fashionable" rules, but therapy. In fact, a few decades back, the cosmetics industry joined forces with the American Cancer Society to deliver the "Look Good . . . Feel Better" program, enabling patients across the nation to help in their recovery with the aid of professional makeup and hair consultants. It was, and still is, a resounding success.

In *Makeup for Ageless Beauty*, Linda shows how it is possible to navigate successfully the bewildering array of makeup products that are available today, and to choose the right colors, tones, and textures, not as cover-up, but to accentuate the positive and eliminate the negative.

It is no longer the chronological passing of time that is aging; it is how we choose to live our lives, with makeup delivering a powerful contribution. Linda believes, as I do, that only neglect is aging. Follow her steps in these pages, and learn that exciting truth for yourself.

Shirley Lord in my studio.

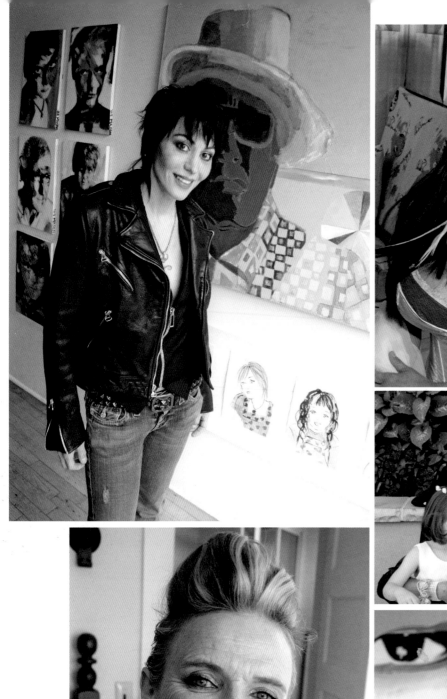
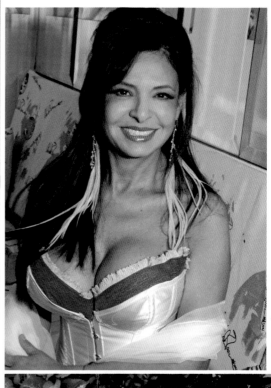
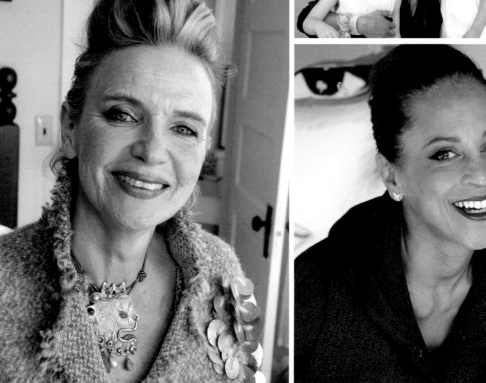
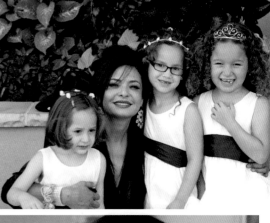

preface

How can women, as we grow older, keep our looks and makeup in harmony with the youthful feelings we have on the inside? How can we use makeup to maintain a healthy glow or feel glamorous without looking as though we're wearing a mask or trying too hard? How do we choose from the overwhelming variety of great products that are available? How do we select and apply colors to best enhance our features?

Makeup for Ageless Beauty seeks to answer all these questions, with the goal of giving you knowledge that will make you feel comfortable purchasing, applying, and—most important—enjoying makeup. You'll find many tips here for improving and enhancing your beauty without becoming a stereotype of an older woman trying—and inevitably failing—to look younger, as well as advice for recapturing the joy of experimentation.

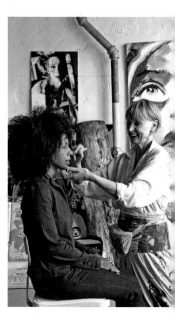

If you're over 40 and you've never felt the desire to use makeup, now is the time to try it! One of my clients, who served as a model for this book, Mimi Oka, never wore makeup until she turned 40. I've noticed that women of a certain age who take care of their hair and clothing and feel good about themselves overall usually look good without makeup but look *great* when makeup is added to the picture. So why settle for just looking good when you can look great?

A commonly held misconception about makeup is that, as we age, we can't wear as much of it. I believe that older women can still wear stronger makeup if they wish, as long as they choose and apply the colors with care. Rarely does one now see caked-on, masklike makeup, not only because the formulations of products have changed but because their quality has improved.

I'm in the fortunate position to have had an incredible career as a fashion and beauty makeup artist, working on photo shoots, fashion shows, and commercials. I've also been privileged to have my own store in New York City, The Art of Beauty by Linda Mason, where I've worked with great women from all walks of life who were interested in making the most of their unique beauty with the help of makeup and where I can apply the vast experience and knowledge I've garnered from my career in fashion and commercial work to the so-called average woman.

For many years, my clients and my publisher had been asking me to write this book. I avoided doing so, however, because I had a conflict: How could I, in just one book, do justice to all these fabulous women I knew? How could I succeed in capturing their inner and outer beauty

Some of the great women who participated in this book (CLOCKWISE FROM TOP RIGHT): Doris Lozada, Doris with her grandchildren, Alva Chinn, Cécile Defforey, and Joan Jett. In the picture of Joan you can see artwork by Cécile (TOP RIGHT), Rina Iwaii, (BOTTOM RIGHT), and me (LEFT).

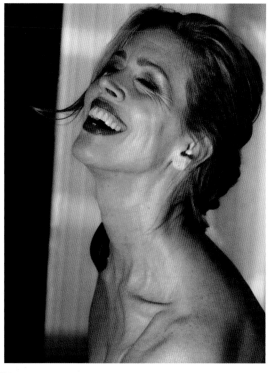

together with their youthful spark, because—yes!—it's still there. Rather than portraying these incredible women as aging inanimate objects, which would have been a terrible mistake, I wanted to capture their real beauty and vitality. And I had another concern: While the contrasts between "before" and "after" photographs are good for shock value (and something I'm guilty of having used in previous books), I wondered in this case what purpose they would serve, apart from perhaps embarrassing the models. Do they really teach readers what to do? So rather than showing each woman "before" and "after," I created photographic sketches that simplify her features and developed one or more makeup "looks" that express who she is and how she feels about herself. The one exception to the rule against "before and after" photos is Silko Coelenbier (please forgive me, Silko), whose makeup is so very subtle that comparing them will clarify the instructions for all the other applications.

Another challenge in doing this book was figuring out how to categorize the makeup looks. I tried organizing them by the models' ages, but that didn't work because many of them can work well on women of any age. I finally settled on overall themes for the makeup applications themselves, starting with Subtle Looks, for everyday wear; Glamorous Looks, for more dramatic effect; and Creative Looks, for those times when you're feeling adventurous and open to experimentation.

A "Mini Masterpiece" makeup compact from my cosmetics line.

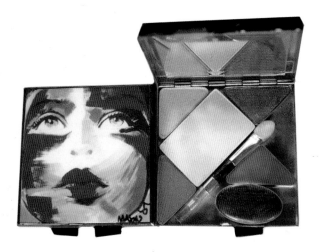

I've known many of the women featured throughout this book since they were in their 20s; others, such as Brooke Shields, Paulina Porizkova, and Anne Bezamat, I've known since they were teenagers. I first worked with Anna Bayle, Alva Chinn, Debbie Dickinson, Gunilla Lindblad, and Lilo Zinglersen in the late 1970s, when they were top models working in Paris. You'll find photos that I took of Susanna Midnight when she was in her early 20s in one of my earlier books, *Makeup: The Art of Beauty,* and she now graces the pages of this one. Other clients, such as the vivacious Doris Lozada (a grandmother and one of the first women to have her own contracting company) and the elegant Diana de Vegh (also a grandmother, who works full-time as a psychotherapist in private practice), kindly accepted my invitation to participate in this project. Each of these women has a personal journey and a story to share about how makeup works for her and expresses who she is. I hope you'll be inspired not just by their looks but by their creative, often adventurous spirits.

Although I've been doing makeup for many years, I've learned new things from working with these women. I feel very honored to have been entrusted with writing this book, which is really about them, and find them more beautiful now than when I began working on it. Their lives, full of joys, trials, and tribulations, have transformed them into sometimes (though not always) less obvious, but quite definitely more fascinating, beauties.

When a face is fixed in time in a photograph and shown close-up on a printed page, every detail is intensified, and readers tend to focus on imperfections such as wrinkles and blemishes. But as we all know, a woman's face is just a small part of the whole and is more beautiful when it's animated with expressive movement. As a woman gets older, she hopes that her life has become richer, which may mean she'll have visible frown lines, or that if she's worried it will be more obvious; but it's also true that if she's happy and radiant, that will be more obvious, too. It's a woman's allure, and the feelings she projects, that are important; she will never be a fixed entity, a mere face seen in close-up on a page. As we age, makeup can become an important expression of who we are. Makeup has the power to make us feel better about ourselves, too, a means of letting the world know that we're enjoying life and are happy. This is what *Makeup for Ageless Beauty* is all about.

I've worked Debbie Dickinson (OPPOSITE) and Brooke Shields (BELOW) since the early days of their modeling careers.

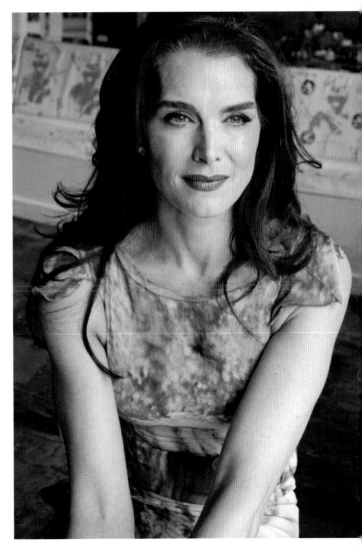

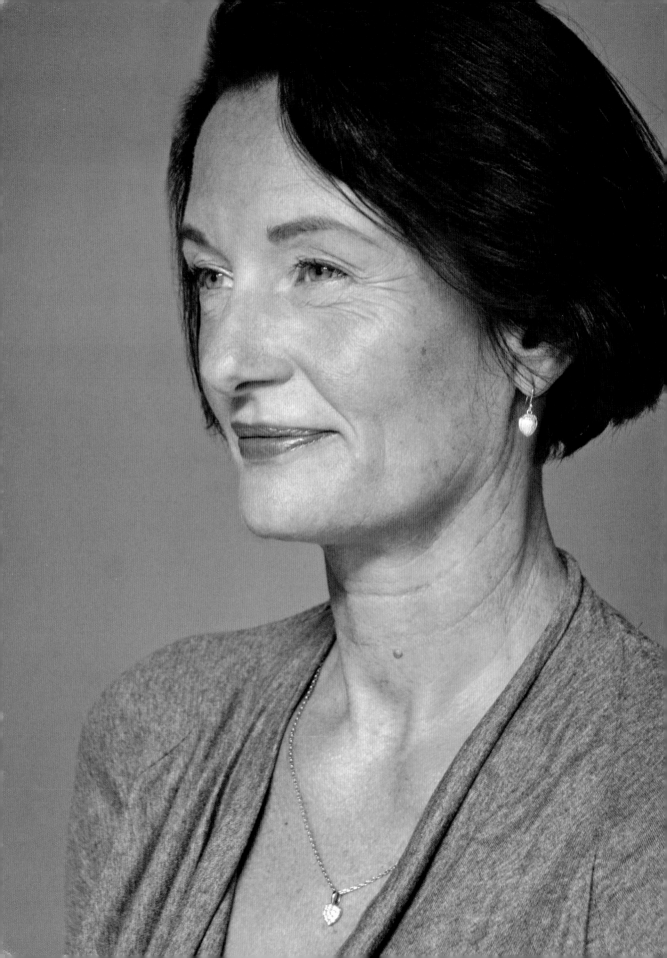

1. before you make up

As one ages, one's skin changes too, becoming drier and yellower in tone, often with red or brown patches. If you're fortunate enough to have great bone structure, then the inevitable wrinkles, fine lines, and sagging skin may not be as obvious and may take longer to emerge. For some women, wrinkles bother them the most, while for others it's the loss of elasticity. For yet others, it's absolutely everything that falls short of perfection. For all women over 40, achieving an even, smooth makeup application requires first and foremost a great skincare regime, so it's impossible to start talking about makeup without first talking briefly about skin.

Lilo Zinglersen in a subtle makeup for every day that highlights her natural beauty. (For more on Lilo, see pages 148–149.)

taking care
of yourself—and your skin

Although your skin's primary characteristics—color, texture, and tone—whether good or bad, are determined by your genetic inheritance, there are three critical ways to take care of your skin and improve its appearance.

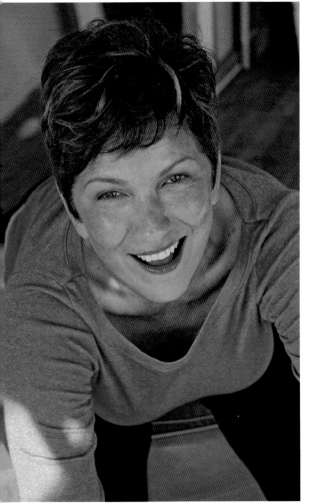

sleep: a nightly facelift

Overscheduling, stress, and hormonal changes are just a few of the reasons that many women over 40 find it challenging to get enough sleep, and they know all too well how a lack of sleep can affect how they look. When you don't get adequate rest, your body secretes extra cortisol (a stress hormone) in order to cope, and this hormone breaks down skin cells. If I'm physically and mentally worn out, I simply must get my requisite seven hours of sleep, which makes a big difference to the freshness of my skin and the bags under my eyes.

diet: feeding skin well

On the positive side, fruits and vegetables have antioxidant compounds that can fight damage caused by the elements (too much wind and sun) and lack of sleep, and the essential fatty acids found in foods such as fish and nuts help nourish skin and keep it looking plump. Some women avoid alcohol because they find that it dehydrates their skin and causes (or aggravates) puffiness.

Mimi Quillin is a Pilates instructor who works out several times a week, including taking two days of ballet class. (For more on Mimi, see pages 102–103.)

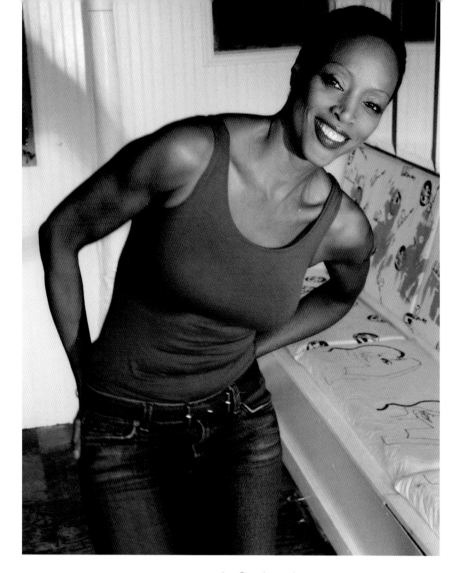

Every morning model Coco Mitchell does Sun Salutations, a set of twelve yoga moves in continuous flow. She calls them her "God Salutations" and uses them to build strength and flexibility as well connect to her spirituality. (For detailed information about Coco's look, see page 162–163)

exercise: a youthful glow

A healthy diet and lots of sleep can help keep skin looking great, but only regular exercise can give you a beautiful, youthful glow and help maintain your energy level. I myself have a very simple exercise regime: I live in New York City and I love to walk to and from my shop and wherever else I need to go, whenever possible. If I really need to get in shape, I swim every morning, something I love to do.

The women featured in this book have their own favorite methods of exercise. Mimi Oka (see page 150) does cycling marathons. Pilates instructor Mimi Quillin's creative and athletic work life certainly plays a major factor in her beauty and makeup routine, and she credits exercise with helping her look her best. She makes sure to drink lots of water and eats a healthy diet. Does she wear makeup to do Pilates or work out? "Yes," she exclaims, "the trainers are so cute!"

cleansing aging skin

No matter how much you like the soap you use to wash your body, it will inevitably dry out and sensitize your skin as you age. Instead of washing your face with soap, use a good cream facial cleanser that's devoid of harsh chemicals such as benzoyl peroxide (meant for acne-prone skin) and glycolic acid, perfume, and artificial colors. Make sure you have a gentle cleansing program in place before you begin experimenting with new moisturizers, creams, and makeup.

Cleansing is a must every evening and sometimes in the morning, though in the morning dry skin may only need a splashing with warm water or wiping with a nonalcoholic toner. For acne-prone skin and enlarged pores, there are special cleansers that can be used once weekly for more in-depth cleansing and exfoliating; alternatively, a facial mask suited to your skin type could replace the exfoliating cleanser.

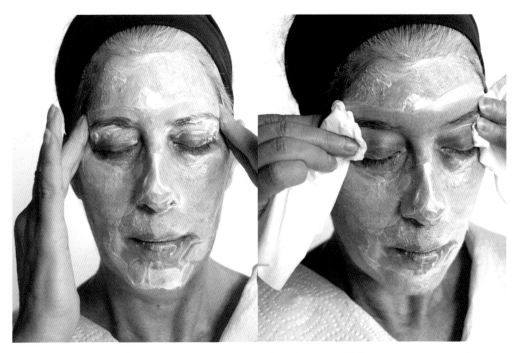

Every evening, start by removing your lipstick, then taking off your eye makeup with an oil-free eye-makeup remover before lightly massaging your face with the cleanser.

Gently wipe off the cleanser with a facial tissue, and then rinse with water or wipe with a cotton ball soaked in a nonalcoholic toner. Don't brutalize your skin during the process; be gentle.

choosing and using
moisturizers

As one ages, the choice of products can be overwhelming, as is the ever-evolving landscape of ingredients that promise to forestall the aging process. You also may find that moisturizer alone isn't enough, or that the products you've been using for years just don't work anymore and might even start irritating your skin, causing redness, or worse, aggravating a pre-existing condition such as rosacea. It helps to define your skin type and your specific skin issues (see a dermatologist if necessary) and then consider the following options.

moisturizer: daily moisture and protection

The first lotion or cream a woman usually uses is a daily moisturizer.
A good moisturizer not only softens, protects, and moistens skin,
but it gives foundation staying power. For a woman over 40, daytime
moisturizer, which has a light consistency and should include sunscreen
to protect against ultraviolet rays, has a different role than a night cream.

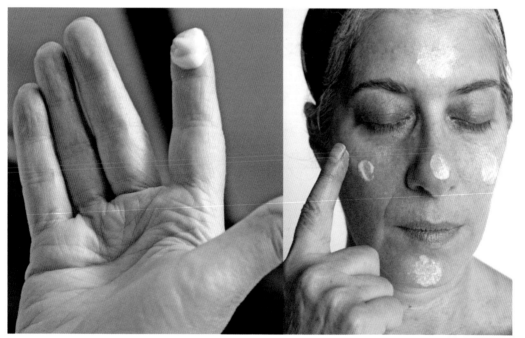

This is all the moisturizer you should need.
Distribute it over your face by dotting it on—
don't forget the nose—then blending it in evenly.

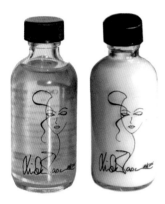

Almond oil (LEFT) and daily moisturizer (RIGHT). I use both products, applying a little oil just to the driest parts of my face (around my nose and between my brows) in the morning, right after I've splashed it with warm water. I apply my moisturizer just before I apply my base.

oils: softening severely dry skin

Almond and jojoba are the two oils with the qualities nearest to those of your own natural skin. Both absorb easily, leaving skin silky but not shiny. Almond oil is one of the least greasy oils and works really well to eliminate flakiness and to soften the skin. While you shouldn't use almond oil if you have nut allergies, it's a good choice for anyone who has difficulty finding a moisturizer that doesn't irritate them or feels that their skin needs a break from more active products. Jojoba oil is a little heavier than almond oil but is still easily absorbed.

To blend oil into your skin, place your fingers together, apply a little of the product to their tips, then apply. You could also dot a little oil down the center of your face, which usually needs the most massaging, and quickly blend outward with your fingertips.

night creams: improving texture

When looking to improve the texture of your skin, you can try one of several varieties of night cream. There are formulations that stimulate new collagen growth, thus encouraging more rapid cell turnover; those that help the skin retain moisture and elasticity and protect against free radicals that break down collagen; or those that encourage various enzymes to repair cell DNA.

anti-wrinkle creams: cell renewal

The cosmetic ingredients that are supported by the most evidence for slowing down the advance of fine lines and wrinkles are retinoids (such as tretinoin, a.k.a. Retin-A) and the vitamin C family (L-ascorbic acid and some of its derivatives). Vitamin A and retinol (a pure and active form of vitamin A) are quite commonly found in over-the-counter products; the prescription-strength products include Retin-A. Active ingredients deriving from this form of vitamin A encourage rapid cell turnover, and different studies have shown that they improve the skin's own ability to retain collagen, increase the amount of new collagen formed, and diminish age spots. The downside to these products is that, for many women, both retinoids and vitamin C creams are too strong, and those with sensitive skin react to them with more sensitivity, flaking, and peeling, and are unable to continue using the creams for the amount of time that's deemed necessary to see results (eight to twelve weeks). This problem can sometimes be counteracted by alternating the cream with a milder nourishing night cream and gentle massages with jojoba oil.

Another ingredient found to be effective in anti-wrinkle creams (as well as for decreasing blotchiness) is niacinamide, which is a naturally occurring form of vitamin B_3. Though niacinamide hasn't been tested as frequently as vitamin A, evidence shows that it can stimulate the production of the body's natural moisturizers, allowing skin to retain more moisture and reducing fine lines, irritation, and redness. Products containing niacinamide can usually be tolerated by more sensitive skin.

eye creams: reducing puffiness

The cream I find women have the most difficulty choosing is their eye cream. Often these products make puffiness worse, and the only way to find out is to try them. Use them sparingly, trying them in the morning as soon as you get up if they don't work for you in the evening. Some are made specifically for daytime and should have an almost immediate effect by reducing bags and dark circles. Eye creams you apply at night repair and prevent further damage around the eyes; retinol, alpha-hydroxy acids, copper, and vitamin C actually work under the skin to stimulate collagen growth and are common ingredients in this type. If you have sensitive skin, it's all the more important that you look carefully at the strength of the firming ingredient contained in your eye cream. Common firming ingredients are caffeine, alcohol, retinol, alpha-hydroxy acids, copper, and vitamin C. Caffeine and alcohol temporarily dehydrate the skin, making it appear taut. Common darkness-inhibiting ingredients are vitamin K, kojic acid, and hydroquinone.

Alva's skin is so radiant, smooth, and even it's difficult to believe that until ten years ago her beauty regime consisted solely of taking off her makeup with cold cream and washing with soap and water. Her regime now includes moisturizer and night cream. (For more on Alva, see page 114.)

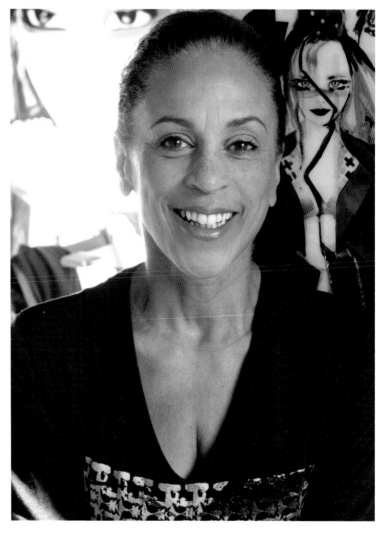

starting a new regimen

Cécile takes care of herself by walking every day, wearing sunscreen, taking vitamins, and getting plenty of fresh air, which she believes is even more important to her beauty regimen than exercise.

When starting new creams, it's best if you can begin using them individually, allowing an interval of a couple of weeks between the addition of other new products to make sure that they don't cause any allergic reactions or irritation. Unfortunately, sometimes you can't get the maximum benefit of a skincare regime other than by using a complete product line, and then I advise starting them together.

Mimi Quillin (see page 102) uses a complete skincare line for her regime. Every morning she cleanses her face with a botanical cleanser and rinses with water. Then she applies a lightweight moisturizer with SPF-15 sunblock. In the evening she uses a gentle eye makeup remover, then the botanical cleanser, and applies a night cream that's heavier than her morning moisturizer. Three times a week, before applying her night cream, she applies a vitamin C–based anti-wrinkle product from the same product line, and sometimes an eye cream to counteract puffiness.

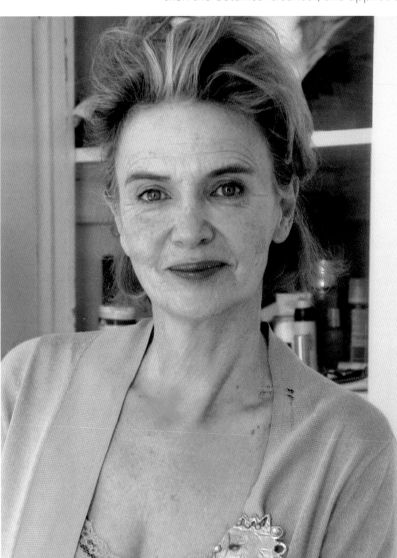

grooming

Regardless of your preferred method of hair removal—tweezing, waxing, threading, or some combination—shaping brows and eliminating facial hair will give your face a visual lift and keep the attention focused on your beautiful look.

long facial hairs

The appearance of long facial hairs really bothers me, so I keep a watchful eye out every morning for these strays, which are easy to pluck out if you can see them. More difficult to deal with is the thicker moustache growth that women tend to get as they age. I've tried quite a few things to get rid of mine. I can't stand waxing, not just because it hurts, but because I read that it can contribute to lines forming above the lips (though I have yet to confirm this correlation), so I do a combination of cutting and plucking, which I feel results in a more natural growth. I pluck out as many longer stray hairs as I can stand in the corners of the mouth and right under the nose, and a few on the chin. Then I take a very small pair of Tweezerman facial hair scissors and, placing the round side against the skin, trim the rest. Threading can be done in these areas too. I do not cut the fuzzy hair growth down the sides of the face. I recommend that it be waxed, although I find it easy and painless to pluck.

A small pair of Tweezerman facial scissors. To remove hairs inside the nose or to trim moustache hairs, put the round side to the skin and cut.

shaping eyebrows

Eyebrows make the defining difference to a face, especially when hair color and brow color are different, so I zero in on them right away.

As one ages, the beginning of the brows tend to sink down, and it becomes necessary to pluck under this area to give a visual lift. To treat the frown lines that sometimes occur between the brows, keep the skin there especially nourished and moisturized; then try to counteract the results of any furrowing by tweezing that area. Removing the light fuzzy hairs that tend to grow on the brow bone is a great pick-me-up, even if they're lightly colored, as they tend to bring down the eyes, making them appear to droop.

If you can stand the pain, waxing gives a precise brow line but isn't as precise as threading. I tend to steer away from waxing, which I find too painful. I can judge my target better with tweezing, so for my brows I pluck the odd unruly gray hair but pay attention to make sure that removing it won't leave a gap. Tweezing gives you more possibilities for shaping brows, and you can give yourself a more natural look and less defined line.

To begin, lift the outer end of your eyebrow up with one finger, then slip the tweezers underneath and quickly pull out the small hairs underneath in the direction of their growth. This will lift the brow in the correct area (see below). If you're nervous about changing your eyebrow shape, this will just give them a quick clean up. You don't need to remove many to have an effect. If you need to remove hairs from between the brows, or from beneath the beginning of each brow, proceed carefully, as women often overpluck this area. Removing just two or three hairs can make a big difference.

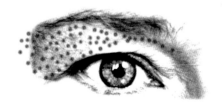 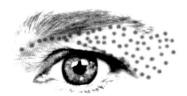

The areas beneath and at the beginning of the brows that require tweezing.

OPPOSITE PAGE: To maintain their shape, Dana Roc has her eyebrows professionally waxed and cut every two weeks. (For more on Dana, see pages 92–95.)

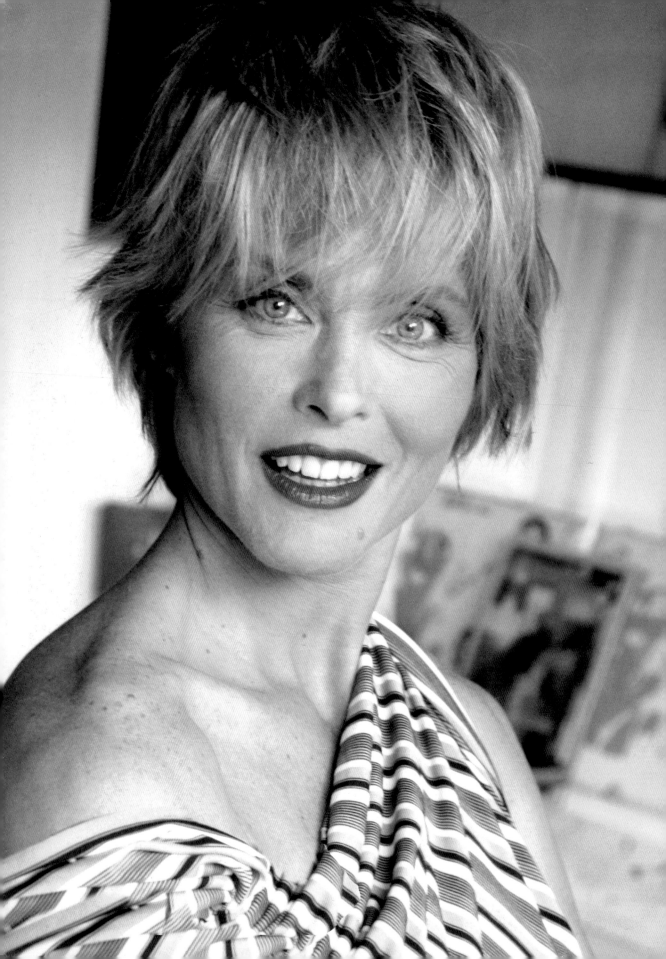

2. preparing the canvas

The goal of this book is to help women apply their makeup beautifully and express themselves creatively. To be able to achieve the best results, your "canvas" needs to be as smooth and well-prepared as possible, and for most women this requires using base, and perhaps concealer, to cover up those pesky problem areas. Not every woman needs to apply these products heavily every day, but from time to time you may feel the need for extra coverage to deal with some of the problems common to aging skin. In this chapter we also take a look at another essential: enhancing the shape of brows with color, which I've included instructions for here because they're such an important part of initial makeup preparation.

Kim Alexis in a look that accentuates her blue eyes (see pages 96–97 for details).

base

Your base makeup, sometimes referred to as *foundation,* is the first step after proper skincare in preparing the canvas that is your face for a full makeup application. There have been many advancements in base products in recent years, making the number of choices a little overwhelming. Cream bases, once heavy and thick, are now smooth and lightweight, which allows them to blend easily with the skin's natural oils. There are also incredible long-lasting translucent gel bases that can be worn alone or under a more opaque product. The textures and shades of liquid foundations are much more natural than in the past.

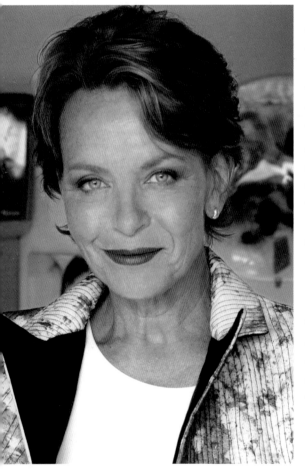

I warmed up Christine De Lisle's facial skintone to match her body tan using a golden shade of liquid base.

I find that, for many women as they age, base is the most important part of makeup, and it's great when they feel so comfortable wearing it that it becomes an intrinsic part of their look. Throughout this book I explain what kind and color of base each woman is wearing so that you can decide whether you like the effect. You'll notice that I've often used a mixture: it could be a gel with a concealer, or it could be a liquid base plus a little cream base plus concealer. I prefer this approach rather than just a flat blending of one product.

When shopping for a base, there's no better way to assess its color than by applying it to your inner arm. If you're planning to wear a powder with it to make the finish matte and longer lasting (see page 38), then you must apply that powder on top of the base. When shopping, don't be afraid to ask the salesperson to examine your inner arm in daylight, with the base applied to it, and to take out your powder if you have one to try over it. If your powder makes your base darker or heavier in any way, then the base isn't a good choice for you, unless you also intend to purchase a new powder.

You'll see examples throughout this book where, as a result of the model having a tanned chest, I chose to deepen her face color using a darker base. In addition to trying the darker base products on your inner arm, it would also be great if you were able to try it on a patch of skin on your jawbone or neck; then, if you wanted to try two qualities or shades, you could test that out on both sides of your jaw. Although a sheerer product may look lighter or darker in its container than one that's more opaque, once blended, the more opaque one will more closely resemble the actual color of the product.

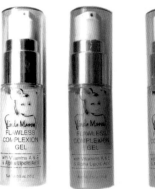

Gel base/minimal coverage: A gel base is very lightweight and will give a smooth, matte finish with light coverage. Unless you have flaky skin, which it will accentuate, it's the perfect product for women who don't like the feel of wearing a base or for those in a hurry who like a clean look. It can be used on its own or under a base. Because gel bases dry quickly, they should be applied and blended quickly. Currently only a limited number of shades are available.

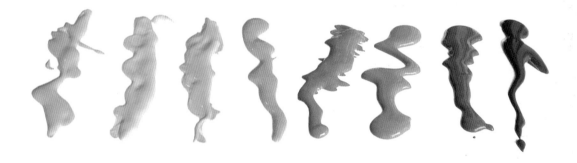

Liquid base/moderate coverage: Some liquid bases are sheer, while others offer more coverage. You can apply these with your fingertips or a damp sponge. Place the fingers together and apply a little of the product on the tips of the fingers and blend. Or dot a little down the center of the face, which usually needs the most coverage and smoothing out, and quickly blend outward with the tips of the fingers. A sponge allows you to blend the product imperceptibly, then to go back over the areas that need a little more coverage, such as your nose or redness in your cheeks. The shades of liquid base used in the book are, from left to right: very pale, very pale with a yellow undertone, light beige, warm beige with a yellow undertone, tan, warm golden, very dark with a red undertone, and very dark neutral.

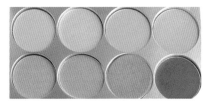

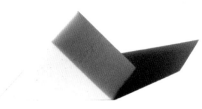

This type of sponge is good for blending liquid and cream bases. For fine, even coverage using a liquid base, you can use a damp sponge, which is gentler on the skin and more economical, because it absorbs less product.

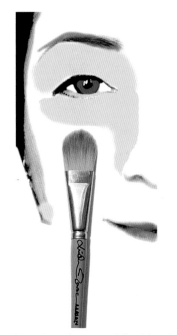

A base brush is good for blending cream base, especially in limited areas, using its flat side. This illustration shows where it's best to use the brush to apply your cream base.

Cream base/maximum coverage: Although a cream base offers a heavier, silky coverage and more of a finished look, you'll still need to apply concealer if you have undereye circles or other imperfections. On certain types of skin (usually finer skin, and on women who don't use night cream), cream base tends to sit on top of it and look too heavy. The colors of cream base used in the book are, from left to right and top to bottom: pale, light beige, light beige with a yellow undertone, medium beige, medium beige with a yellow undertone, warm beige, warm beige with a red undertone, and dark.

A note on mineral makeup: I don't generally use this product on clients who are over 40 because it imparts a slight allover shine to the skin, which is great when you have no sagging, but will accentuate it if you do.

Correcting yellowing or dullness: Even if you have red patches here and there, your skin tone can still yellow or dull as you age. Diet, overall health, and sun exposure all have a cumulative effect on the skin's appearance.

For women with a tanned complexion, brightening the skin means warming it up with either a tinted moisturizer or a warm golden base. This is also the case for dark-skinned women, who are advised to use products with a golden glow or a red undertone.

For very pale skin, a tinted moisturizer will often dull the skin by making the face darker than the neck, taking away from the beauty of the natural skin color. I look at the neck and chest of a client to see if the face is darker; if it is, I use a very light liquid base that I blend in until it becomes invisible, which lightens and brightens the skin. The new gel bases work well for this too, as long as you can find one that's slightly lighter than your skin tone. In some cases, I actually use white base on very pale skin usually that of a redhead to achieve this effect.

concealer

Concealer is usually applied over base makeup to selectively increase coverage to areas that need evening out or visual balance through lightening or darkening. It can be tricky to apply when trying to avoid accentuating any puffiness, crepiness, or lines, especially under the eyes, so its consistency and application are both very important. I like a cream concealer that doesn't have much shine to it, which I apply to small areas with a brush, then dab with my fingertip to make sure it's well blended before powdering very lightly.

Concealer should have more coverage than the base you're using, even a cream base, so when in doubt, go with a shade of concealer that's slightly lighter than your base. If it turns out to be too light, you can always dab a little of your base over it: It's better to have areas that need concealer be a little lighter, particularly around the eyes, where it can serve as a backdrop for eye shadows. The one exception to this would be if you have light rings around your eyes (see Finn O'Gorman, page 126). They are usually from being in the sun wearing sunglasses.

Before concealing a problem, it's important to first look at its underlying causes and the condition and texture of the skin to assess whether any additional moisturizing or other treatment may be needed.

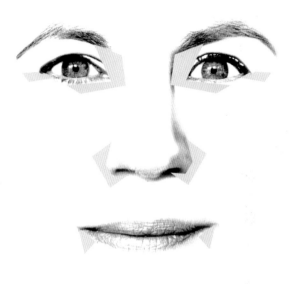

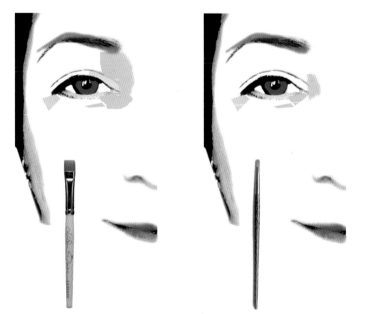

ABOVE: Areas of the face that typically need concealer.

LEFT: To apply concealer, use firm brushes whose size matches the size of the area you're working on. Remember to use all three areas of the brush—tip, side, and edge—when applying and blending.

redness

Very often redness can be found on the nose and cheeks, though the chin can also become redder than the rest of the face. Redness in these areas can be dealt with in a variety of ways, depending on the type of base you like to use and the condition of your skin. If you're wearing a heavier base, then it may cover everything. If not, go back over the areas where the redness is showing with a cream base or concealer. A concealer provides more coverage than a cream base.

If you need to, you can also try a special product used for scars that tends to last longer because it's drier and more opaque than concealer (see page 34). This product should be the same color as your base or slightly lighter. If you don't like heavy coverage, use a face gel or lightweight base to even out the skin lightly, then apply the product sparingly to those parts of the face that need it and blend well.

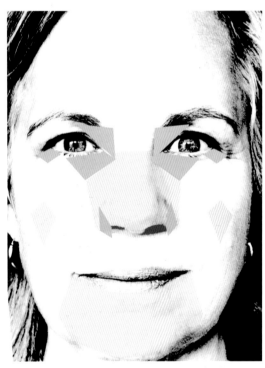

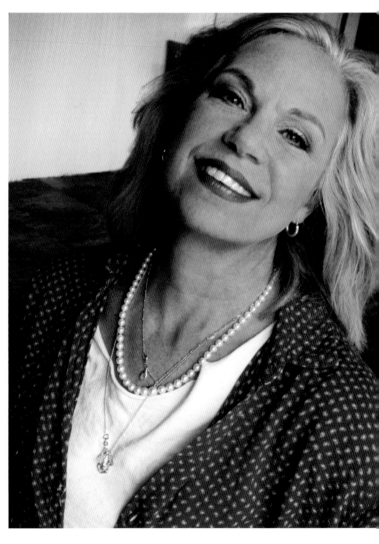

For Joan Elizabeth Goodman I applied a lightweight base to her entire face. Then I used a cream base on the areas that needed more coverage such as her nose, chin, and areas on her cheeks where she had some darkening. Lastly, I used a cream concealer to lighten and give even more coverage to the inner and outer corners of her eyes and the sides of her nostrils.

red, dry patches

Sometimes problem skin requires you to become a detective of sorts. One day a scaly redness suddenly appeared under my eyes and in the center of my forehead between my eyebrows that created thin wrinkles in the inner corners under my eyes. I had been washing them with soap for a few weeks before the redness appeared (I had been too lazy to use my eye makeup remover) and imagined that to be the cause. I massaged the areas gently with a dot of jojoba oil, and this made a big improvement. Then a doctor told me it was contact dermatitis and prescribed a cortisone cream. At first I was horrified, as this seemed to only crinkle my skin and dry it out further. Then I started alternating the cortisone cream with the jojoba oil and the redness improved. I disinfected my eyeglasses with alcohol and changed my diet, because my condition seemed to get worse after I had eaten certain foods the previous evening. Because of the redness and dryness under my eyes, I was unable to use my concealer in that area. However, I did continue using it in the inner corners of my eyes, next to the nose, which helped me look less tired.

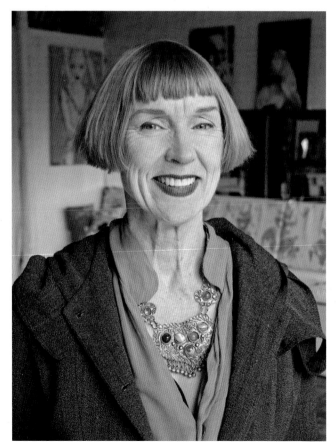

Apply concealer only to these areas

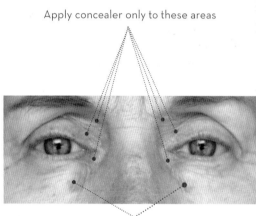

Avoid these scaley areas

To conceal area of redness around my eyes, I selectively applied concealer to avoid the dry, scaly patches.

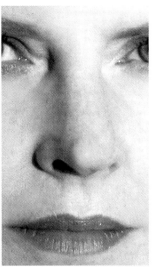

scars

There are a couple of special coverage products on the market that work well on scars, such as Dermablend. Just make sure that the shade you choose is lighter than your skin tone; if it's darker, it will deepen the scar.

First apply a minute amount of the product with a small concealer brush to any brown edges you may have around the scar; then apply it to the scar and around any redness. If there's flaky skin around the scar, try massaging it lightly first with jojoba oil on a cotton swab.

A scar before (LEFT) and after the application of a product formulated to minimize the appearance of scars and other pronounced flaws.

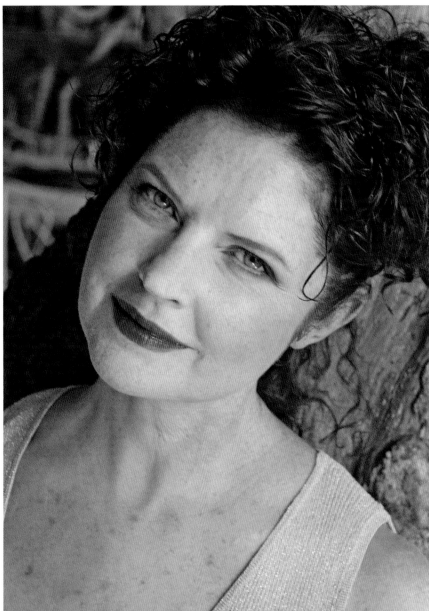

Margie Martin, a visual artist, regards the scar on her nose, which was caused by cancer, as a "scar of courage."

brown marks

Brown marks on light skin should be treated similarly to scars. Because these marks are darker, the product should be lighter to lighten them. To apply it, tap it on the spot to blend it in with your fingertip. As with redness, you can dab on a little base makeup over the mark once you've covered it if you feel it's too light. Once you apply powder, everything should blend together.

For darker skin, you can start by applying one base color to the face, then a lighter base or concealer to darker areas. (If necessary, you can add a darker base or concealer to the lighter areas.) An application of colored powder will give you an even finish.

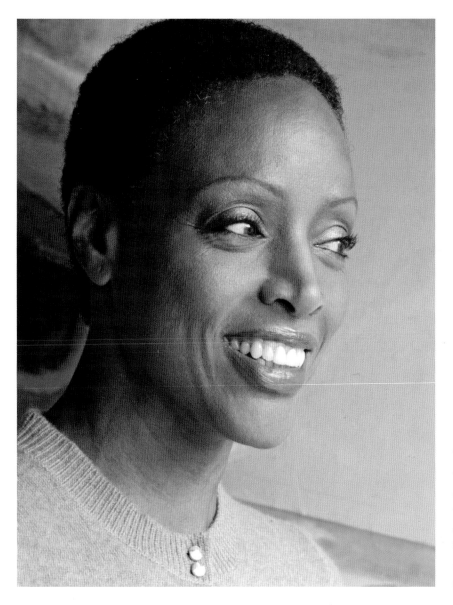

To even out Coco's skin tone, I applied one color of base to her entire face, then a lighter base over darker areas and a darker base over the lighter ones before finishing with powder in a warm color.

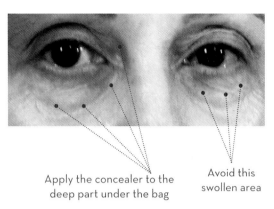

Apply the concealer to the
deep part under the bag

Avoid this
swollen area

Apply concealer to the deep part of the
undereye bag and to the inner and outer
corners of the eyes, avoiding the puffy "bag."

undereye bags

It's possible in some instances to use too much
concealer, and undereye bags is one of them. It's best
in this case to apply concealer selectively to the inner
and outer corner of the eyes and avoid putting it all
over the undereye area.

If you have bags under the eyes marked by a
darker line directly under the area that's puffy or
swollen, it's better to use your base lightly under your
eyes, then to go into the indented line beneath the
pouchy area with your concealer on a small brush.
This type of condition is often paired with deepness
in the inner corners of the eyes, where you can also
apply concealer to diminish the dark, cavernous
appearance (see below). You should always go lighter
with your concealer, as you can always pat on a touch
of your base color over it to blend it in.

sinking eyes

Over time, the darkening and thinning of the skin in
the inner corners of the eyes makes deep-set eyes
appear to sink even deeper. To counteract this effect,
lighten your eyelid with concealer or a cream base,
paying special attention to the inner corners, where
the eyes tend to "sink" the most. Sometimes the area
under the eye is just too heavily lined, in which case
it's better to forgo concealer there. Also see "drooping
lids" on page 56.

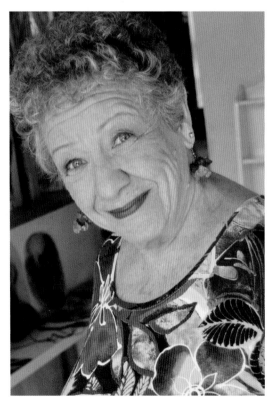

I didn't use concealer in the areas beneath
Phyllis Molle's eyes to avoid emphasizing
the lines there. (For more on Phyllis, see
pages 164–167.)

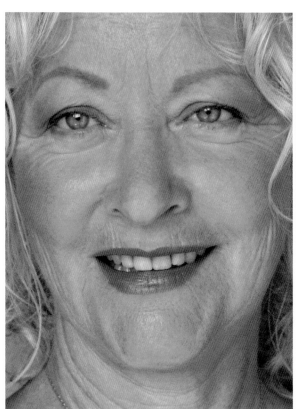
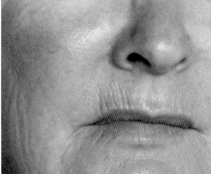
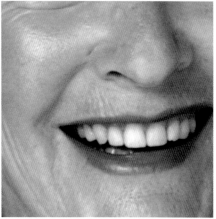

pucker lines

Pucker lines around the mouth are common in older women, especially smokers. Line fillers are available for use before applying your makeup, though these generally work better for finer lines. Massaging above the upper lip from time to time with almond or jojoba oil helps prevent dryness and softens the skin in this area so that your makeup won't become too cakey. If you need concealer in this area, make sure you apply it sparingly so it won't sink into the lines. Once you've finished applying your makeup, check well—if it looks cakey, roll a tissue around your finger, stretch your upper lip, and rub the area lightly, which will eliminate any excess makeup or flaky skin.

I minimized Finn O'Gorman's pucker lines with careful base and concealer application. To keep lipstick from bleeding, use matte lipstick and outline with a soft pencil liner, then powder the outline with translucent powder.

BELOW: Lighten these areas around the mouth with concealer.

drooping mouth

If your mouth droops at the corners, one trick to lighten these area is to add a touch of concealer—and don't forget to smile!

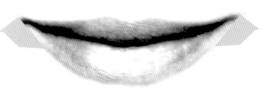

powder

One key thing to remember when both shopping for and applying your products is that any area to which you apply shine will be accentuated and become more prominent. This rule goes for both concave and convex areas, so don't apply shine or iridescence to any areas where there's sagging, drooping, wrinkling, and unwanted sinking. When skin is young, smooth, and plumped up, we can pretty much use any type of product without creating unwanted effects, and most women in their 40s still have free rein. But as we move into our 50s and 60s our options become more limited, and we need to assess the areas of the face that attract the light and if they are unflattering minimize them with powder.

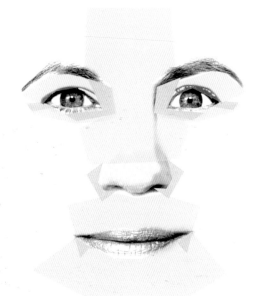

Minimize shine by applying powder to these "danger" areas: the nostrils, the tip of the nose, around the mouth, and on the chin. These are also areas where you should check for redness and use concealer first if necessary and avoid products with shine or shimmer.

A great translucent powder is very useful. Even if you like a healthy glow with a slight shine, it's still wise to make sure that the areas around the nostrils, chin, nose, and any other sagging or overly prominent spots are kept matte with powder once any redness is hidden with concealer or base. Apply powder to these areas using a large, firm, clean eye shadow brush. (This isn't the same as merely dusting powder over your face loosely, which won't help "fix" your makeup.) If you just want certain areas matte, press the powder on with a large eye shadow brush; for a finished matte look, take a cotton powder puff and press in the powder over your entire face, then give it a final overall dusting with your large, soft finishing brush.

Another way to fix your makeup and remove excess powder is to go over the skin with a damp sponge once you've powdered it. For darker skin, I like to use translucent powder, then sometimes add another powder with more color on top.

To achieve a bronzed effect without using a deeper shade of foundation or tinted moisturizer, you can dust a bronzing powder on the cheekbones and lightly around the face.

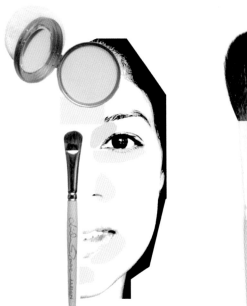
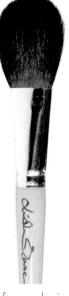
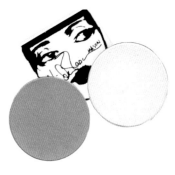

Translucent powder gives a matte finish and "fixes" your makeup in place; darker powders give more coverage to deeper-toned skin.

Use a large eye shadow brush—one that you reserve for exclusive use with powder—to press translucent powder into small areas that need it the most. Use a face finishing brush to dust on a light layer of any shade of powder. For a long-lasting finish or before a photo shoot, use powder puffs to press on powder in larger areas of the face.

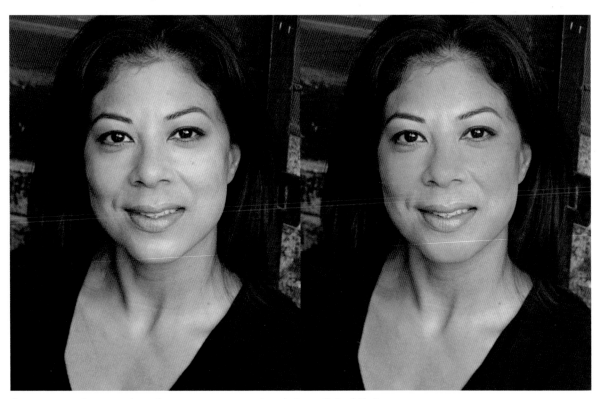

Bronzer used sparingly enhances a warm, natural glow. Grisel Baltazar before (LEFT) and after applying bronzer. (For more on Grisel, see pages 144–147.)

contouring

As a rule, I don't recommend that women do a lot of contouring because it can make a face look too masklike and transform it to the point where identity is obliterated. But there are some products and techniques that, when used subtly, are helpful for gently accentuating bone structure.

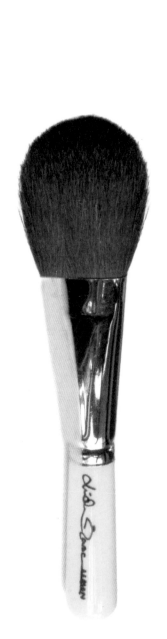

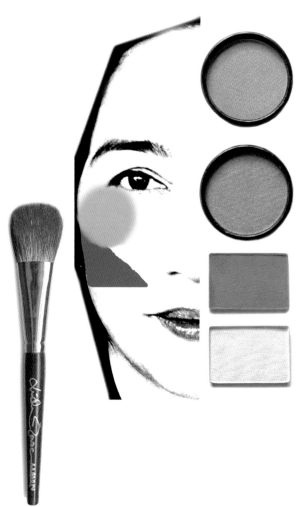

Lighter contouring powders, which can be used alone for their soft color or as a highlight or mixed with other blushers, give a very soft, natural shine. Darker and brown powders should be used low on the cheekbones, but not too low—just on the lower part of the bone itself. Apply these powders with a contour brush, which is firmer than a blusher brush and a great choice for when you need more control over the placement of shading.

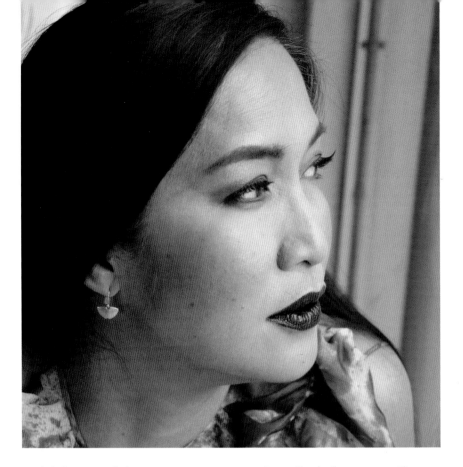

I did a some light contouring on writer Anna Bayle (see page 118), who's more voluptuous than in her modeling days, a plus for her skin, which is more filled out and therefore has no sagging or wrinkling. As a result, it was very easy to do a little contouring with cream bases: a darker one to slim down specific areas of her face and neck and accentuate her cheekbones, and a slightly lighter one to bring out the eyes and smooth the skin. I also blended a medium beige concealer over the lids and under the eyes before finishing with a translucent powder.

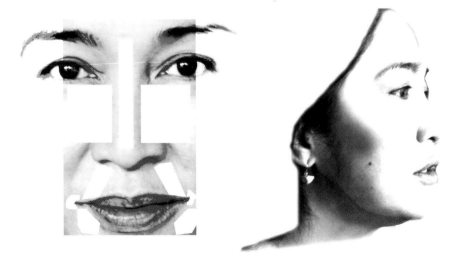

To define the jaw and minimize jowls, gently blend either a deeper shade of base with a base brush or a matte brown powder with a contouring brush around and under the jawbone. As one ages, contouring under the cheekbone generally becomes less necessary, as this area tends to sink, but it can be very flattering on a wide or round face.

reshaping and
accentuating brows with color

Brows are generally a women's most eye-catching feature, and there are many ways to accentuate them, depending on your desired look. I talk a bit about grooming eyebrows in Chapter 1, "Before You Make Up" (see page 25), but beyond removing excess hair, brows can become problematic as we age: they tend to sprout gray hairs, become discolored, wiry, and unruly, and may thin out to the point of disappearing completely. Heavily or severely penciled brows can draw too much attention, so I prefer a more subtle approach, using a mixture of products to achieve a natural appearance.

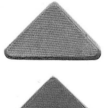

Colors: The colors of shadow or pencil I use on brows depend not just on brow color but on hair color as well. A blond pencil is very good for light hair; if you have dark hair and are wary of using pencil, you can use this color first, then blend in a darker color once you have the line that you want. For powders, I use gold to counteract gray; a soft beige mushroom to lightly define a natural-looking brow of any color; gray to mix in with the browns; dark brown for a more sophisticated look; and black powder for very dark hair.

On my own brows, I pencil in the areas that have become sparser using a blond eyebrow pencil. Depending on the tone of my hair at the time, I may lightly brush in a warmer color (with either the spiral wand or, if I want more definition, the angled brow brush). If I've just had my hair colored, I tend to apply color a little stronger than normal.

Eyebrow powders and pencils are available in a wide range of colors, from light blond to black. Always start with pencil, using a light color if you're unsure about where to apply it, then soften with a spiral brow wand. If brows need more definition, apply brow powder with an angled brow brush.

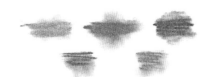

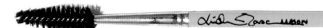

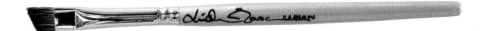

Application: When using pencil, apply it with light feathery touches to the entire brow or to the skin in the sparse areas. Then, using a brow brush, soften the lines and blend the penciling in with the hairs of the brows. For a natural-looking brow, it's best to use first pencil, then powder.

A spiral brow wand and an angled brow brush.

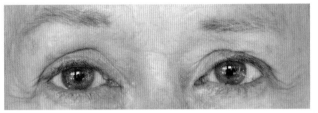

Brushing powder onto your eyebrows with the brow wand will color the hairs lightly. When brushing in the color with the angled brow brush, create a natural appearance by using the flat side of the brush, or define the brows with more shape and sophistication using the tip.

If you're in doubt about to what to do with the shape, thicken the brows where they begin, making sure they're arched lightly, and then taper them off. If there are no brows, start where the natural brow begins, directly above the inner corner of the eye. Don't overemphasize the arch. Instead, aim for a natural line by lifting it slightly at the point just above the outer corner of the eye.

Many times brows don't need to be thickened, they just need a light filling in with a pencil. To naturally deepen the brows, dust them with the side of your angled brow brush to color just the hairs. To give your brows more definition, dab the angled edge of your brush into your shadows, place the edge of the brush with the longest side facing inward onto the beginning of the brow, and draw the brush over the roots. Make sure that the apex of the brows is well colored and tapers off, following the descent of the brow.

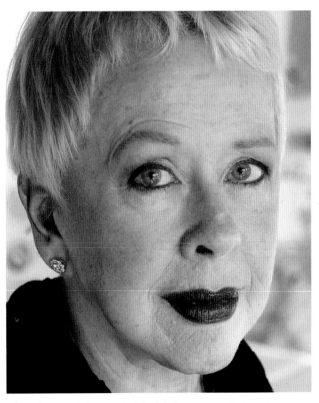

The shape of Diana de Vegh's brows were perfect—starting at the inner corner of the eye, then arching above the outer corner; they just needed some strengthening with blond brow pencil. (For details on this look, see pages 116–117.)

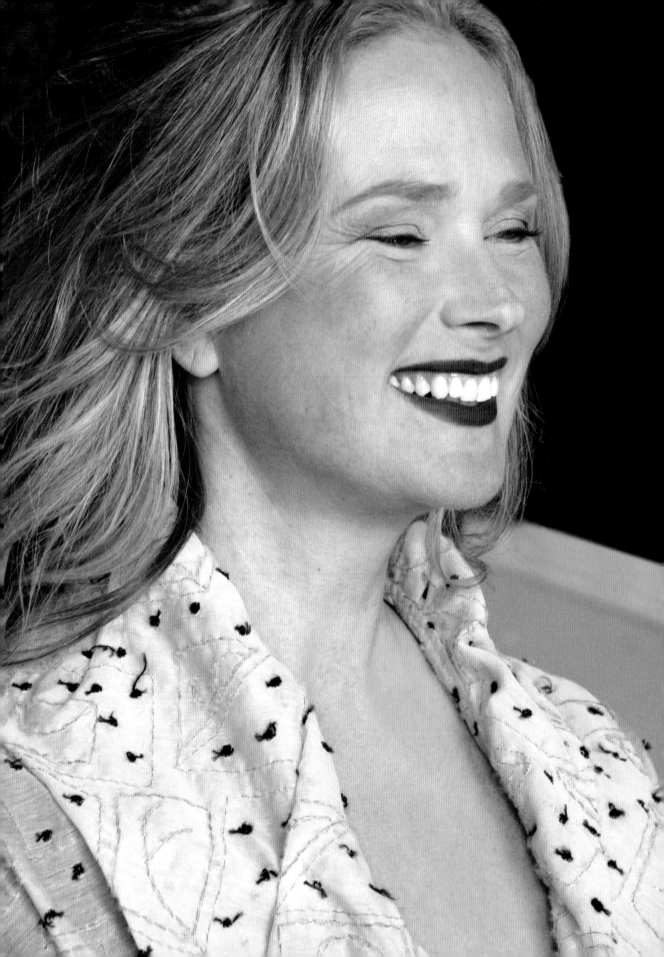

3. applying and playing with color

Color is the fun part of makeup. Even when you're using neutrals like brown or gray, there are so many shades that choosing and applying them is still about working with color. One of the wonderful things about makeup is that you don't always have to be practical about it; you can buy a product or color for the sole reason that you want to try it. In this chapter I talk about colors for eyes, cheeks, and lips—the order in which I discuss them reflects how I apply them—techniques for using them, and some new ways of thinking about color.

Nancy DeWeir Geaney in a colorful look that reflects her creative personality. (For more about Nancy, see page 160.)

reevaluating
your look

For many women, turning 40 can be a major aesthetic turning point, a time to examine their approach to makeup. This reaction is often prompted by catching a glimpse of yourself in a family photo and not liking what you see. You might also feel like you're stuck in a rut, or insecure about whether you're wearing too much makeup, or that the way you're applying it may be unintentionally aging. Those who have never worn makeup and have great skin and strong features may start feeling a little washed out and not as attractive, especially in photos. A fresh approach to makeup can help get you out of your rut, giving you the tools and confidence to rediscover yourself and redefine your image.

RIGHT: Diana evaluates a look that I designed for her. (For details, see pages 116–117.) OPPOSITE: A guide to the terms used throughout this book for the elements of the face when describing where and how to apply color.

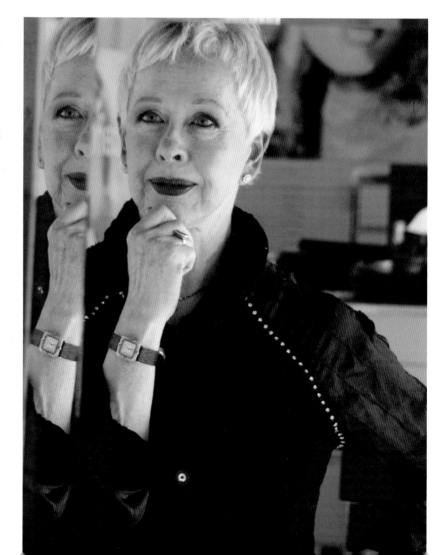

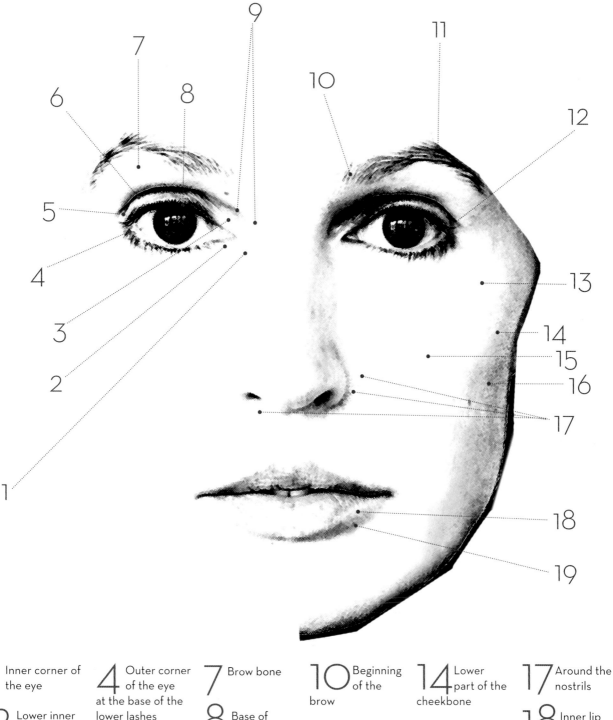

1 Inner corner of the eye

2 Lower inner corner of the eye next to the rim

3 Upper inner corner of the eye

4 Outer corner of the eye at the base of the lower lashes

5 Outer upper corner of the eye

6 Eye crease

7 Brow bone

8 Base of upper lashes

9 Upper inner corner of the eye next to the nose

10 Beginning of the brow

11 Apex of the brow

12 Lower inner rim

13 Cheekbone

14 Lower part of the cheekbone

15 Apple of the cheek

16 Under the cheekbone

17 Around the nostrils

18 Inner lip line

19 Outer lip line

color for eyes

When we talk about eye makeup, we're really talking about three different areas and their products: shadows for lids; liners for upper and lower lash lines; and mascaras and false eyelashes for lashes. Within these categories are several different kinds of products and application tools you should become familiar with, if you haven't already. The options for applying shadows and liners are endless, and in this section we'll focus on how you can adjust your application to keep up with the challenges of mature skin.

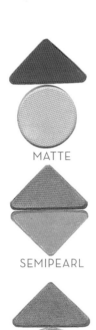

MATTE

SEMIPEARL

PEARL

IRIDESCENT

Eye shadow finishes range from matte (no shine) to iridescent (the most shine).

eye shadow

I think eye shadow is the most fun part of applying makeup—it's where you really become an artist. It allows you to transform the shape of your eyes as well as enhance or complement your eye color. Depending on the application, eye shadow can make your eyes look bigger, wider, or sleeker, and create looks ranging from subtle to glamorous to playful, dramatic, and eccentric (see chapters 4 through 6).

Mineral eye shadow. Mineral makeup, which is usually sold as a loose powder, is made from finely ground minerals. Because it's all natural and doesn't contain any of the chemicals or preservatives found in most forms of makeup, many claim that it's better for skin. Its fans love its light, long-lasting glow.

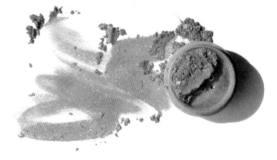

RIGHT: The most flattering browns have an undertone of color. From left to right: brown-pink, brown-red, brown-yellow, and brown-orange.

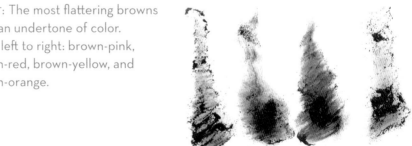

Mini-eye shadow brush. A firm, sable-haired brush is great for blending eye shadow or pencil in small areas. Firm brushes also allow you to first press the shadow into the eyelid before blending so that more of it will stay put.

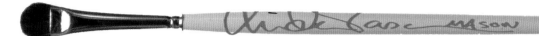

Small eye shadow brush. A small brush is ideal for blending eye shadows in small areas.

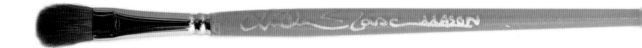

Large eye shadow brush. A larger, slightly more flexible brush suited for dusting color over a large area of the eyelid.

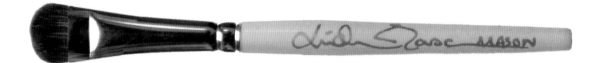

Wide shadow brush. A firm brush that's used to press or blend color into eyelids, it's also great for pressing translucent powder into specific areas of the face.

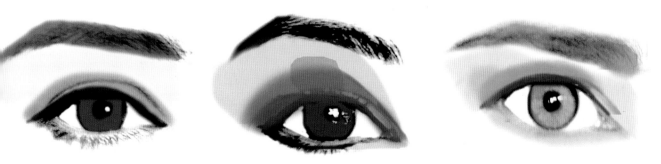

Eye shadow is so versatile that it's easy to open yourself up to its endless creative and color possibilities, from soft neutrals to vibrant brights.

making iridescent shadows work for you

Generally speaking, it's safer for women over 50 not to wear iridescent eye shadows because they accentuate eyelid crepiness (fine surface wrinkling) and other wrinkles, but there are ways to use them to selectively highlight and brighten your look.

One way is to apply iridescent shadow at the base of the lashes in the inner or outer corners of the eyes. If you have a very smooth lid, you could also gently brush on iridescent shadow using a soft, large brush either over the brow bone (directly under the eyebrow) or down the center of the lid. These placements would also work for lighter shades of mineral shadows.

There are many different degrees of iridescence or pearlesence, and testing a color on the back of your hand can give you a fairly good idea of how it will look on your eyes and the degree of shimmer it contains. Sometimes a slight shimmer can make an eye shadow easier to blend, which makes it useful as a base for applying matte shadows.

Iridescent eye shadows have a tendency to scatter easily, so use a small firm brush (such as the mini- or small eye shadow brush shown on page 49), pressing into the base of the lashes or the inner corners of the eyes so that the shadow won't crumble and fall.

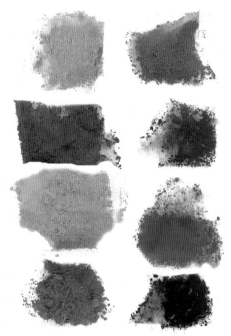

Matte eye shadows.

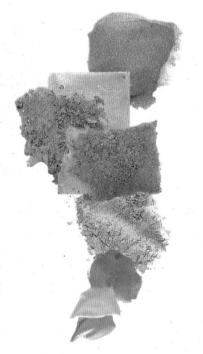

Iridescent eye shadows.

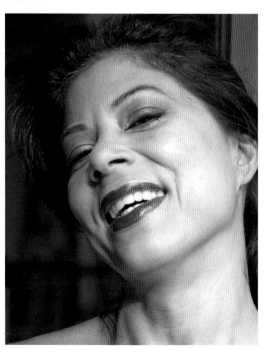

LEFT: Grisel looks great with iridescent shadow blended over her smooth lids. OPPOSITE: In this look, Joan Jett's silver iridescent shadow is positioned at the base of the upper lashes in the inner third of the lid— a safe place for most women 40 and over to apply it.

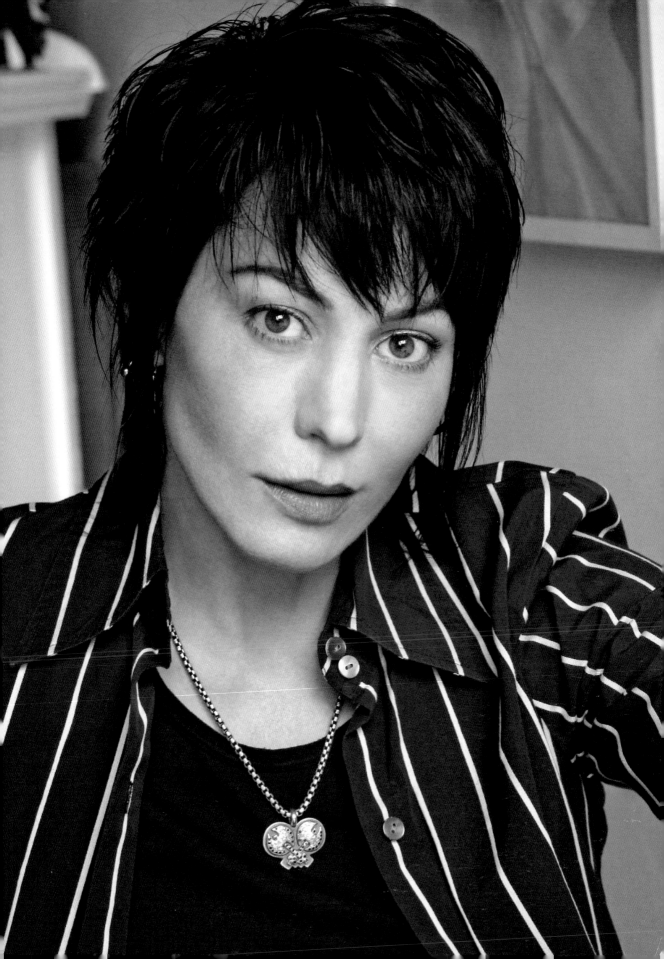

eye liner

Eye liner brush. This is a great brush for achieving a fine line with gel, cake, or liquid eye liner.

Carol Alt wearing Audrey Hepburn–style eye liner, which gives the eyes a strong lift. (For more on this look, see pages 124–125.)

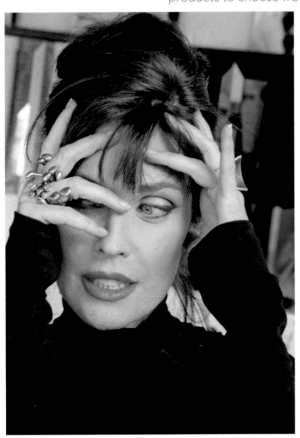

I see many women making the same mistake in applying their eye liner: The majority make it too thick in the center of their lids. This makes the eyes appear larger and rounder, but it also tends to accentuate any downward slope of the lids. After a certain age, it's better to keep liner thinner over the pupil and heavier in the outer upper corners of the eyes, at the base of the lashes.

To apply a fine line, begin at the outer corner of the eye. If you make a mistake or make it too thick, it's less of a problem to correct (this should be the thicker part of the eye liner anyway). Lift the lid up with your finger. Press the liner into the outer corner of the eye and blend it inward, making the line narrower as you apply it. To give the eyes an upward lift, end the line before reaching the center of the lid.

Depending on the desired effect, there are a variety of eye liner products to choose from.

Pencil liner: Pencils are firm and can be sharpened, and therefore are good for getting into small areas and giving you control over your application. Their strong color also works well under shadows.

Gel liner: Gel eye liner is waterproof, and therefore long-lasting. It's great for creating a defined line (you can smudge it too), but you have to work quickly because the line dries fast. Certain colors of gel liner tend to dry out relatively quickly, so if you don't use them frequently, it's better to use cake eye liner.

Cake or liquid liners: The best options for creating a defined line are liquid eye liner, which is sold with either a thin brush or felt-tip applicator, and cake liner, which comes as a solid in its own handy compact and is mixed with water to a paste each time it's used. Both are also easy to remove (with a moist cotton swab) if you make a mistake. I find they're better than gels for crinkly eyelids.

playing with color: colored eye liner

Colored eye liner is a quick, really fun way to add a touch of color to your look. It doesn't necessarily have to be bright; there are many beautiful eye liners with just a hint of color.

I like to use bright liners like red and blue, which may seem like bold choices, but there are more subtle options, such as red-brown or black with a red undertone or fleck of color. See below for other great examples of how to wear colored eye liner.

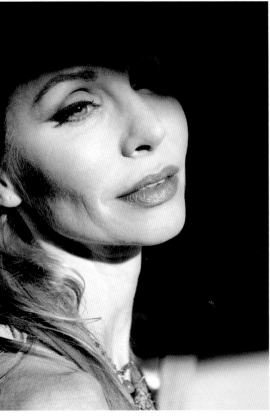

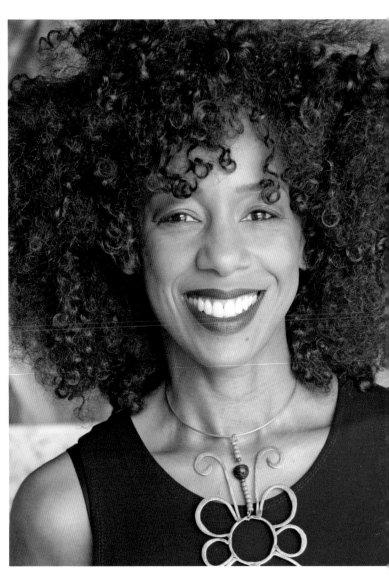

ABOVE: Susanna Midnight wearing strong cake violet eye liner with matte pink lip color. RIGHT: Dana pairs bright blue eye liner with red lipstick. (For more on Dana, see pages 92–95.)

lashes

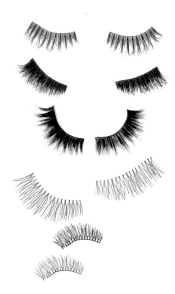

False eyelashes in a variety of styles.

Eyelashes can be enhanced and intensified with mascara, eye pencil, and false eyelashes.

Mascara: Applying mascara is usually the finishing touch to making up eyes. Brown mascara has a slightly softer look than black, which has more of an edge to it. Though I've used black mascara in most of the looks in this book, brown can be substituted in all except for Bibi Lencek (pages 84-85), Brooke Shields (88-89), and Mimi Quillin (102-103) in Subtle Looks; Joan Jett (130-131), Anna Bayle (118-119), and Carol Alt (124-125) in Glamorous Looks; and Coco Mitchell (pages 162-163) and Grisel Baltazar (144-147) in Creative Looks.

When applying mascara, it's best to work the wand in a back-and-forth motion (as opposed to up and down) to get the mascara right into the base of the lashes, which makes them appear much thicker, especially if they're light in color. Another easy fix for thin lashes is to brush in a cream thickener first, then use a mascara with a comb applicator instead of a wand brush.

Penciling sparse lashes: If your eyelashes are very sparse, which is sometimes the case for blonds, or for brunettes with short, straight lashes, it's better to use no mascara at all; for these situations, I recommend just penciling along the lash line to give the appearance of thicker lashes. Lift the eyelid with your fingertip and rub a soft brown or gray pencil into the very base of, or between, the lashes that are there. This will give strength and definition to your eyes better than mascara will, and you may even find you have no need for mascara. If you find that this eye liner comes off under your eyes, then go back in with a small eye shadow brush and press a soft gray or brown eye shadow into the pencil to fix it in place and use translucent powder under the eyes.

False eyelashes: Some women love using false eyelashes, which can be used to create many different types of looks. Light brown false lashes on a light base are sometimes a good substitute for mascara, as are clusters (a grouping of three or four hairs that are glued on individually). If you're wearing temporary false eyelashes, it's better to apply your mascara first so that you can then remove the lashes before you remove your eye makeup and reuse them.

I use several different types of false eyelashes in a variety of looks; see pages 118, 133, and 151 for examples of this. By applying Doris Lozada's lashes after I had finished her eye makeup, I was able to

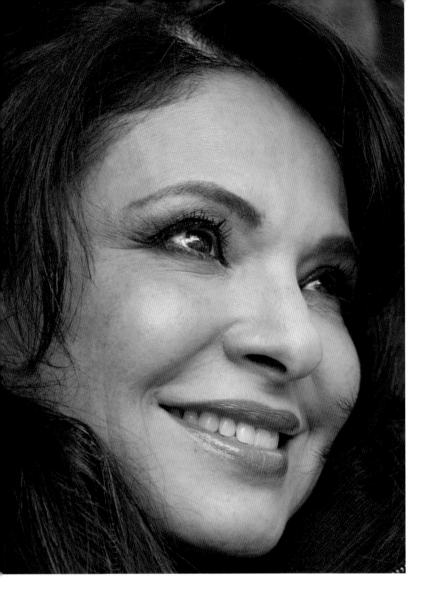

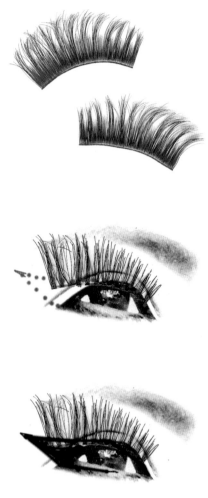

position them starting at the base of the lashes and give her eyes more of an upward sweep by gluing the lashes onto the skin, away from the base of the lashes. If you do this, put your finger under your lashes and blink on them to push the lashes in the right direction—curling upward.

Permanent false eyelashes are glued to your real lashes and fall out when your lashes fall out naturally, and they should be done by a professional. If you wear these, it's probably better not to use mascara on them so they'll last longer.

After applying Doris's eye liner and mascara, I gave her eyes more of an upward swing with a line of false eyelashes whose shape feathered outward.

changing eye shape with shadows and liners

As you read through the looks, you'll find that virtually every one presented an opportunity to enlarge, lengthen, and lift eyes with shadow. Below and on the following pages are techniques that can be incorporated into any look.

drooping lids

For many women, the upper eyelid starts to sag over the eye to the base of the lashes, necessitating a change in the positioning of eye shadows. First make sure that the areas under the brows are well

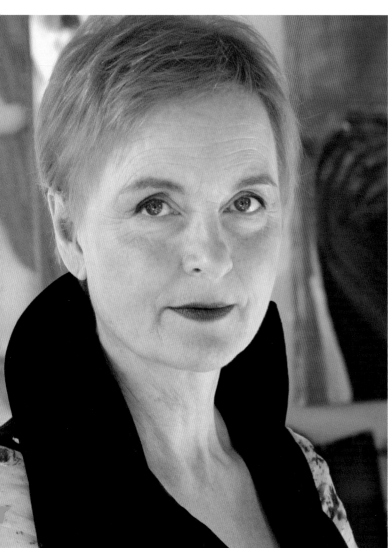

tweezed (see page 25). Give them a visual lift with a touch of a light matte shadow, which emphasizes the high part of the lid just under the brow and also de-emphasizes the fold of the lid that overhangs the lashes. Blending a medium shade of matte shadow from the base of the lashes past the crease of the eye, over the fold, will also help minimize the overhanging eyefold.

If you feel as though the outer edges of your eyes are starting to droop as well, use a soft brown or gray pencil in the very base of the upper lashes to line the outer third of the eye, where the lash line starts to descend.

In addition to blending Kikan Massara's shadow from the base of her upper lashes upward and outward toward the end of the brow, I applied gray pencil there as well. (For more about Kikan, see pages 86–87.)

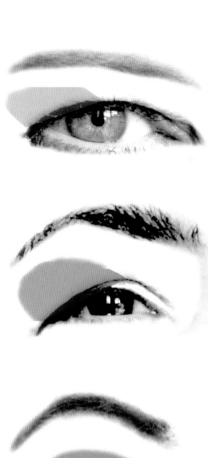

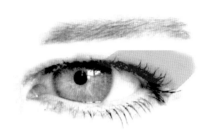

1 This placement lengthens eyes and accentuates an almond shape.

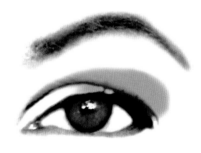

2 Blend shadow up and out to lift the outer corners.

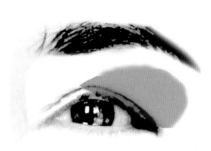

3 Another, more compressed placement of shadow that also lifts eyes at the outer corners.

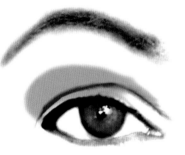

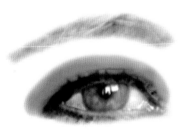

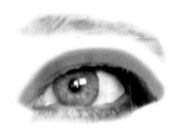

4 If your eyes are widely spaced, you can use this shadow shape to enlarge their appearance.

elongating round eyes

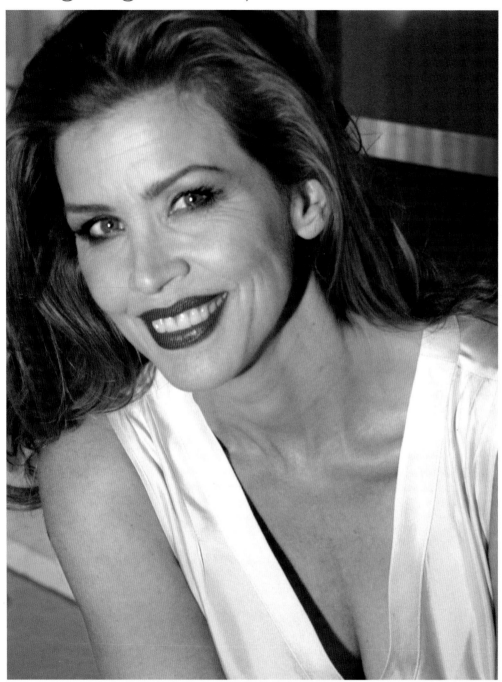

Model Debbie Dickinson in a look that elongates her eyes. (For more details on this look, see pages 132–133.)

The following are detailed instructions for elongating round eyes with eye shadows. This technique will also work for anyone whose eyes are deep-set in the inner corners.

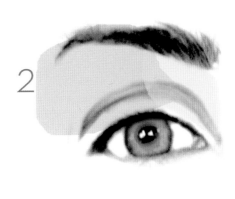

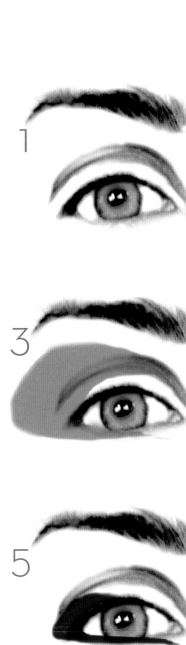

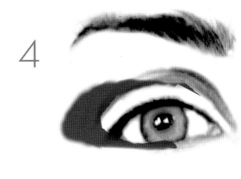

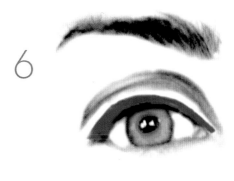

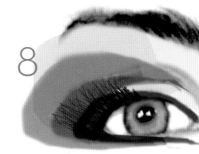

1 Debbie's eye shape before the elongating makeup is applied.

2 With the small eye shadow brush, apply **a pale shadow** to the inner corners of the eyes. With the large eye shadow brush, apply a gentle wash of a **slightly deeper color** from the base of the lashes to the brows on the outer half of the eyelid.

3 Using a small eye shadow brush, lightly blend **a deep matte shadow,** first under the eye, then extending it outward, sweeping it around into the crease, and finally extending it past the crease.

4 With your mini-eye shadow brush, apply **the same shadow more heavily** under the eye at the very base of the lower lashes, then blend it heavily in the crease in the outer third of the eye. Note: This shadow isn't applied under the inner corners of the eyes, which gives the outer corners a visual lift.

5 With the side of your mini-eye shadow brush, blend a **black eye shadow** in the very base of the lower lashes, departing from the lash base in the inner corner and extending to the outer corner. Blend the same shadow in the outer upper corner of the eye from the lashes to the crease.

6 Apply **black or another deep shade of eye liner** to the very base of the lashes.

7 Apply three or four clusters of **medium eyelashes** (or demi lashes) to the very base of the upper lashes in the outer corners of the eyes to lengthen them and give them a natural upward sweep.

8 The finished eye.

creating depth and lift

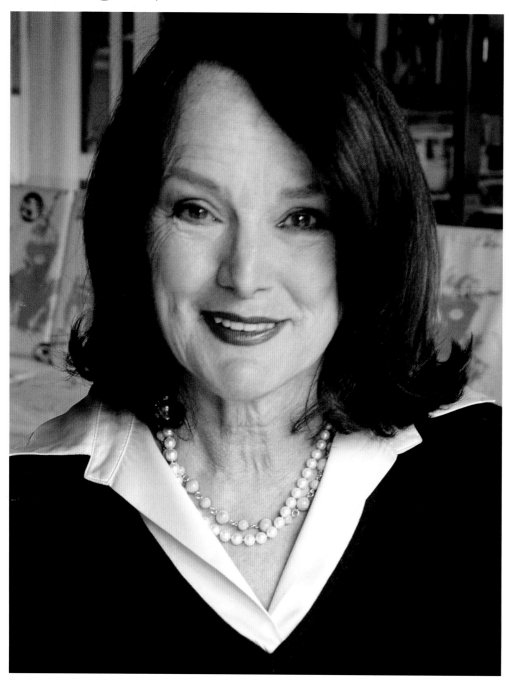

Barbara Novogratz in a layered eye shadow look that gives her eyes a lift and creates depth. (For more about Barbara and this look, see pages 138–139.)

Shadows can be used to create the illusion of depth as well as a visual lift, especially when the area above the upper lid overhangs it, which tends to give the eye a flat appearance.

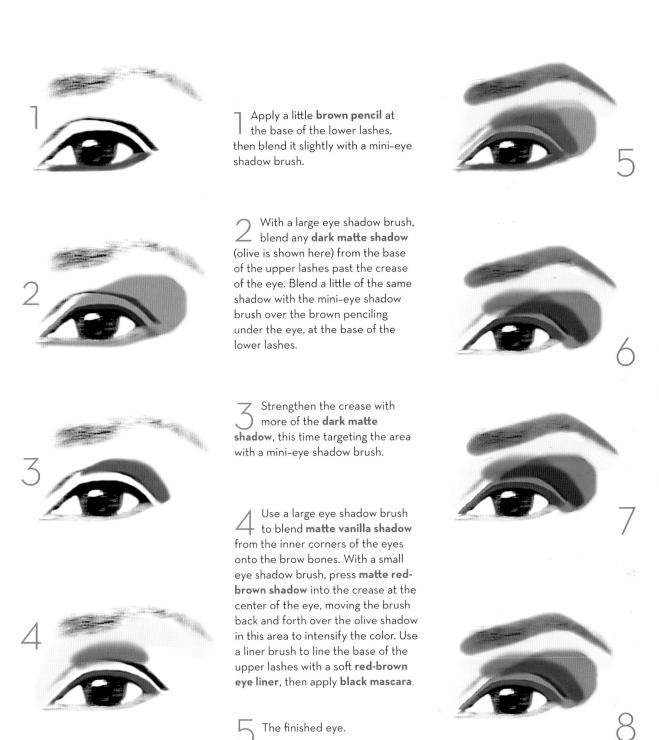

1 Apply a little **brown pencil** at the base of the lower lashes, then blend it slightly with a mini-eye shadow brush.

2 With a large eye shadow brush, blend any **dark matte shadow** (olive is shown here) from the base of the upper lashes past the crease of the eye. Blend a little of the same shadow with the mini-eye shadow brush over the brown penciling under the eye, at the base of the lower lashes.

3 Strengthen the crease with more of the **dark matte shadow**, this time targeting the area with a mini-eye shadow brush.

4 Use a large eye shadow brush to blend **matte vanilla shadow** from the inner corners of the eyes onto the brow bones. With a small eye shadow brush, press **matte red-brown shadow** into the crease at the center of the eye, moving the brush back and forth over the olive shadow in this area to intensify the color. Use a liner brush to line the base of the upper lashes with a soft **red-brown eye liner**, then apply **black mascara**.

5 The finished eye.

6, 7, 8 The same look in three additional colorways: burgundy, violet, and brown.

updating bold eye makeup

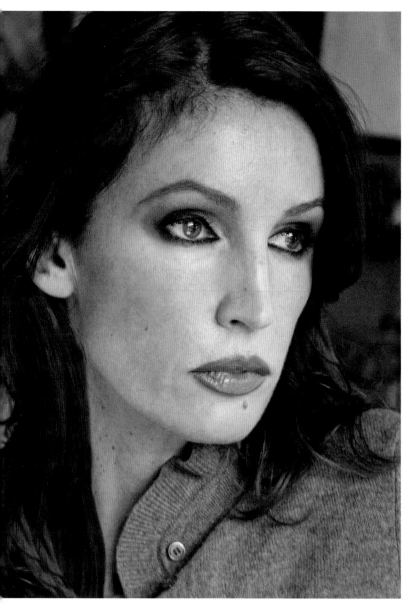

The biggest mistake that women over 40 make with their eye makeup is to apply too much shadow to the inner corners of their eyes. This draws the eyes together, deepens the inner recesses, and makes a woman look more made up overall. These problems are exaggerated when iridescent colors are used. (For guidance on how to use iridescent eye shadow, see pages 50.)

In the sketch at right, I show how I subtly updated model Anne Bezamat's favorite palette of monochromatic browns—adjustments that most women will need to make as they age. The sketch also shows the danger zones of the eye and the products to avoid applying to certain areas.

Heavy undereye penciling or lining can also make a woman look older. The easiest solution is to simply forgo it and strengthen the color on the outer corner of the upper lid to lift the eyes. If you really like this look and are reluctant to give it up because it

For a bold look that isn't heavy-handed or unduly aging, I adjusted the application of matte eye shadows and liner on model Anne Bezamat.

suits your personality, you can apply the liner or pencil less heavily and make a change in their application as well as in the positioning of your blush, as I did for Anne. After a bit of fine-tuning, the brown shadows and undereye penciling look just as great on her as they always had. For a touch of freshness that the right shade of pure color can bring, I added a soft coral blush starting high on the cheekbone, blending it downward, onto the apple of the cheek.

This sketch compares a dramatic shadow and liner look (left) with a more subtle application that still comes across as strong but is lighter and thus less aging (right).

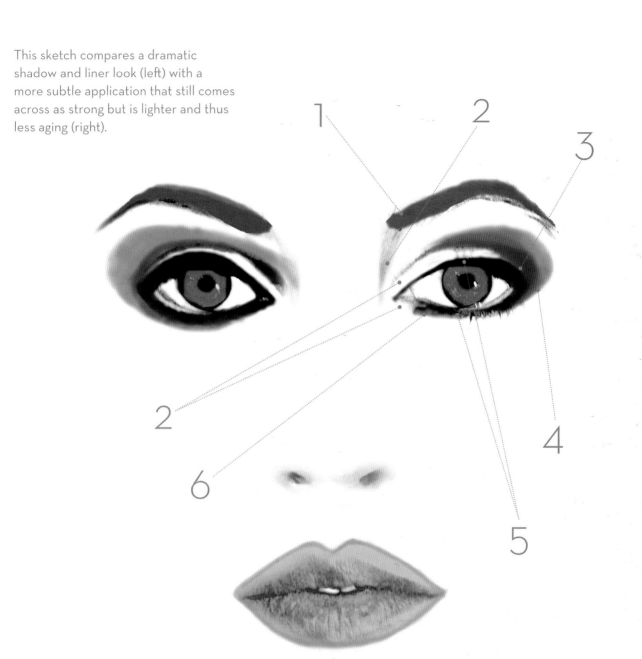

1 Lift the brows here by removing small hairs and avoiding dark shadows and liners.

2 Keep these areas light, but avoid color and shimmer, though you may use a little shimmer at the base of the lashes.

3 Always make the liner and shadow heavier in the outer corner of the eye, after the pupil, where the eye starts sloping downward.

4 Lift the color here.

5 Make the pencil line thinner over and under the pupil at the base of the lashes. Thick shadow or pencil here makes the eyes look heavy and appear to slope downward.

6 Bring the pencil line down slightly, away from the rim of the eye.

the smoky eye in color

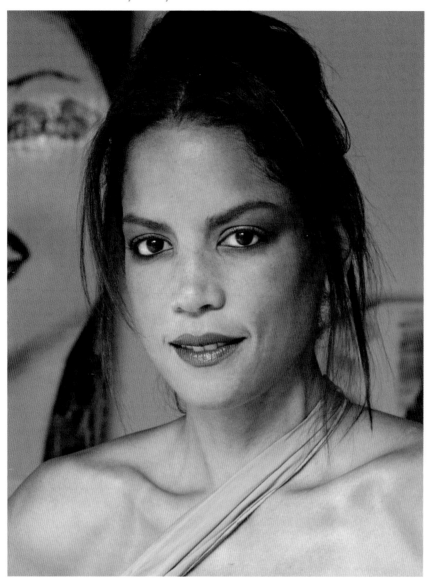

Veronica Webb in a colored smoky eye. For a variation on this look, see pages 158–159.

The smoky eye look has been very popular in recent years, as seen in fashion magazines, on runways, and at red carpet events. When done well, it can make a very dramatic, glamorous statement on women of all ages. This look can be achieved with shadows and liners of many different shades: You don't have to limit yourself to black or brown. At right are detailed application instructions for a strong, smoky eye using black pencil. If you prefer an intense smoky eye with just the color around the eye and no shadow, or a light shadow under the brow, then replace step 3 with a pale eye shadow, or just eliminate that step completely.

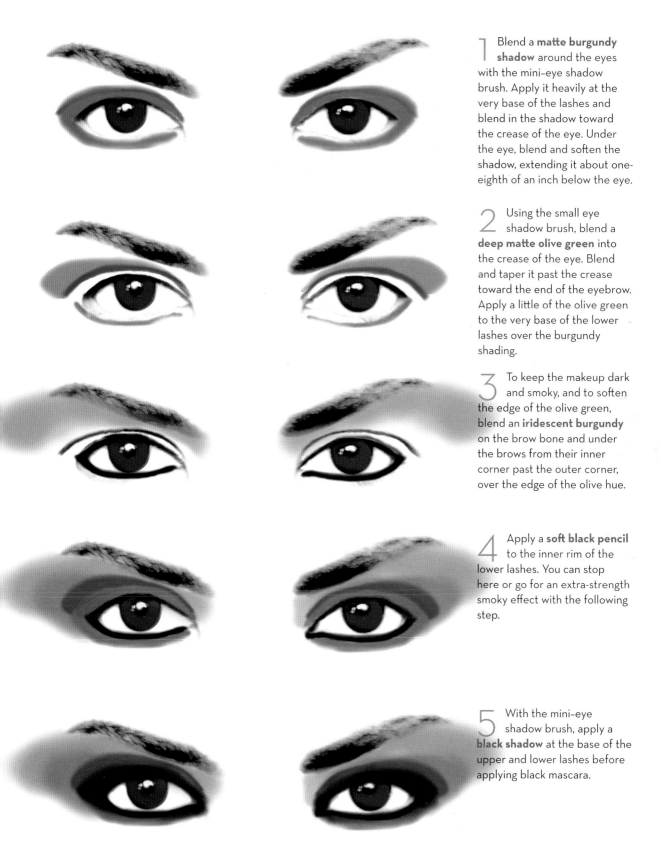

1 Blend a **matte burgundy shadow** around the eyes with the mini–eye shadow brush. Apply it heavily at the very base of the lashes and blend in the shadow toward the crease of the eye. Under the eye, blend and soften the shadow, extending it about one-eighth of an inch below the eye.

2 Using the small eye shadow brush, blend a **deep matte olive green** into the crease of the eye. Blend and taper it past the crease toward the end of the eyebrow. Apply a little of the olive green to the very base of the lower lashes over the burgundy shading.

3 To keep the makeup dark and smoky, and to soften the edge of the olive green, blend an **iridescent burgundy** on the brow bone and under the brows from their inner corner past the outer corner, over the edge of the olive hue.

4 Apply a **soft black pencil** to the inner rim of the lower lashes. You can stop here or go for an extra-strength smoky effect with the following step.

5 With the mini–eye shadow brush, apply a **black shadow** at the base of the upper and lower lashes before applying black mascara.

playing with color: bright duets

One of my favorite ways to combine color is really quite simple—I just pair two colors as a duet and go from there. If you look at Jan Jaffe's makeup below, which is simply two colors layered in the outer corners of the eyes, you can see just how easy it is to give your makeup combinations a boost. I've suggested several makeup duets at right that could work as well as Jan's. Which are you drawn to?

Make a swatch on some paper of your favorite lip color and put it next to the duets and see if they work well together. Then put your lipstick next to the other duets and see if it works better with any of these. If you do buy these new colors, make sure they're either matte or have very little shine to avoid any difficulties you might have with iridescence on aging skin. In this case, you can use color alone to accentuate your beauty.

Jan Jaffe's makeup features two layered eye shadow colors—bright gold and deep peach—with red eye liner. For more on Jan, see pages 170–173.

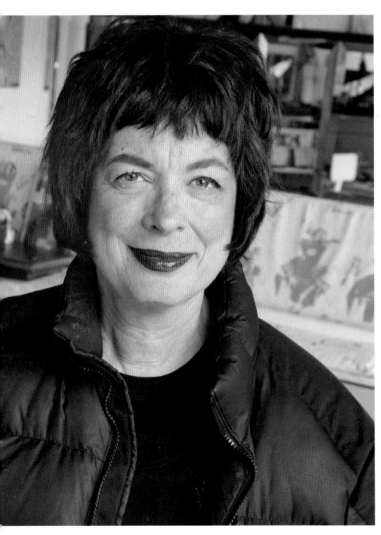

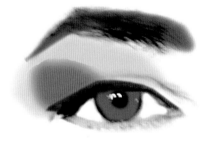

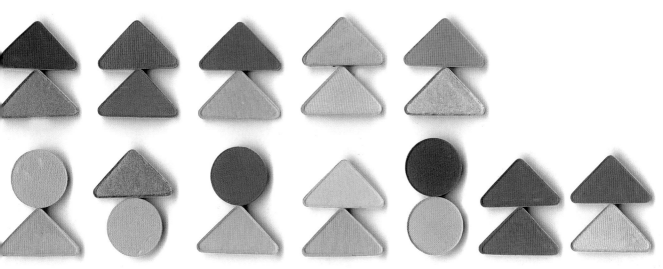

If you prefer a more subtle effect, choose a soft semimatte beige-mushroom color or a matte beige and dust it over the bright colors with a large eye shadow brush to tone them down. Another tip for muting colors: If you have a fairly oily lid, work the bright color into the natural oils and blend them with your finger to leave behind washes of color. Or blend in a cream shadow very thinly, then add a touch of powder to the base next to the eye. Use just a dab of brighter color as a highlight on more muted or neutral shades.

Suggested eye shadow duets to inspire you: Apply the top one over the bottom, but don't cover it completely.

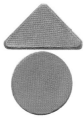

Use neutral shades like these to tone down brighter ones.

playing with color: violet shadows

Violet shadow is a favorite with many women, so it never seems to go out of fashion, but wearing it well is all about attitude. If, unlike Coco Mitchell, you don't feel comfortable in a bold application (see page 162 for a look featuring an iridescent retro 1970s eye), it can look dated or overpowering.

To play it safe with more subtle, beautiful violets, use monochromatic matte shades (see Grisel's look, opposite) or modernize them with a touch of iridescence in a contrasting shade (Susanna's look, below, features a pale green iridescent shade in the inner corners of her eyes). Violet eye shadows range in color from pink tones (perfect for green or hazel eyes and pale skin) to blues (great on dark skin with an olive or blue undertone). For Grisel, the matte violet tint goes just past the crease (not to the brow), making it much easier to wear in the daytime. The iridescent violet shadow is more vibrant and well suited for the evening. Wearing shades of violet with little or no blush makes them fresher and easier to wear.

BELOW: Iridescent and matte violet shades.
RIGHT: Susanna in violet shadow.
OPPOSITE: Grisel wearing matte violet shadow to just past the crease of the eye.

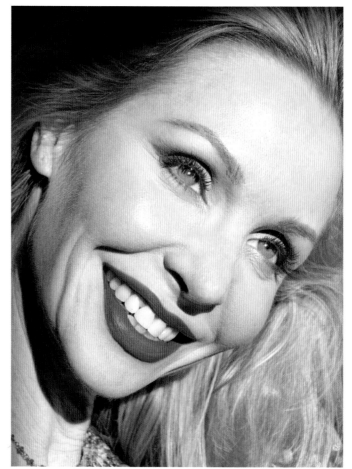

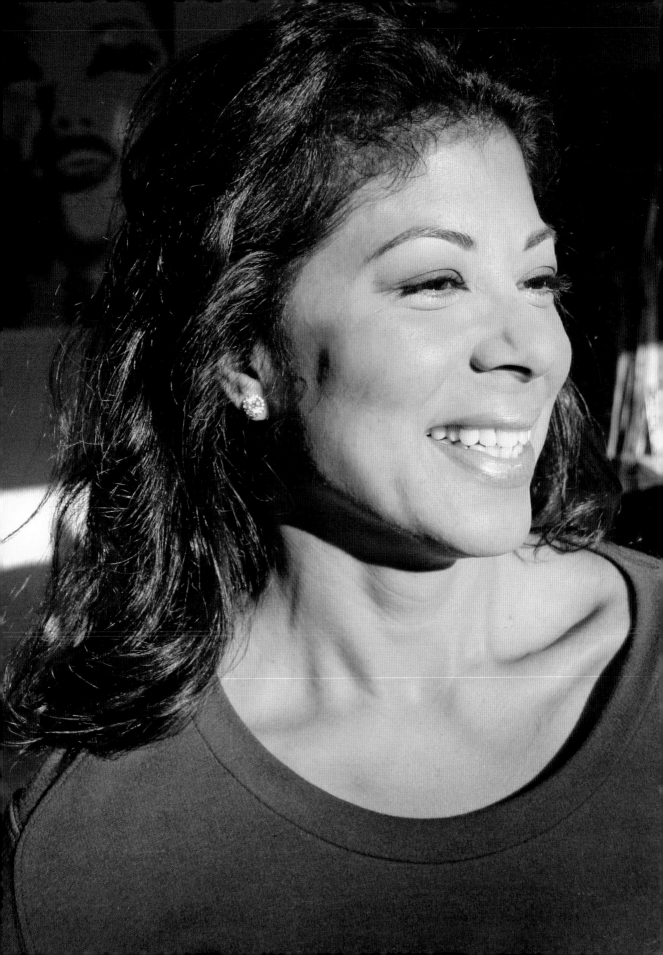

color for cheeks

There are a few different types of blush products, each with its own consistency and finish. As when choosing a base, choose your blush color by testing it on your inner arm if you can't try it out on your face.

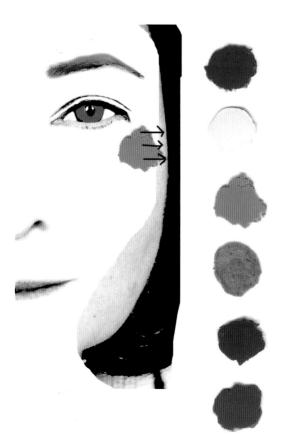

You can only really know how much blush you need after you've finished your eyes and lips, so I recommend that you apply your eye makeup first, then a light application of your blush, followed by your lip color. Then you can assess whether you need to strengthen your blush.

Cream blush: Because cream blush will blend in imperceptibly, it's good for those women who want to achieve a fresh look with very little color. Use your fingers to apply a dot to each cheekbone, blend it outward, then gently tap it on the apples of the cheeks. The colors of cream blush used in this book are shown at left; from top to bottom, they are: dark pink, pearl, light pink, bronze, red brown, and red.

Gel blush: Gel blushes are very similar to creams in that they're also transparent and applied in the same way; however, they need to be applied quickly, as they dry fast and can't be changed once they've been applied, so they're also longer-lasting than creams. To apply, dab a dot onto the skin and blend outward, toward the edge of the face with your fingertips, then tap around the edges of the blended area. Go over the bone under the eyes and, for a fresh look, tap on the apples of the cheeks. This will soften the edges and give a little color to these areas.

Powder blush: Depending on the desired effect, powder blush can either be dusted softly on with a blusher brush or applied with a contouring brush for more precise placement and shaping. Unless you're just applying an overall light dusting of color with a blusher brush, it's always better to blend a powder blush from the outer part of the face inward because its intensity should favor the outer part of the face. If you have good skin, you could use a cream blush during the day, then strengthen it with some powder blush in the evening.

Using the fingertips, blend cream blush in the direction indicated, then tap it lightly on the apples of the cheeks.

As can be seen in the makeup looks featured in the chapters on Subtle Looks, Glamorous Looks, and Creative Looks, powder blushes in colors like orange and lavender can be surprisingly flattering. Start by using them sparingly, as you can always intensify the application.

Mineral blush: Mineral blush usually has a sheen to it. As with any pearlized or shimmery blush, for most women it's best applied to the cheekbones with a blusher brush to give a lift, as opposed to the apples of the cheeks, which can sometimes attract too much light and attention to the center of the face, creating a sagging effect. I recommend avoiding grayish blush colors, which tend to dull the face, and colors that are too heavily pearlized, which emphasize lines and large pores.

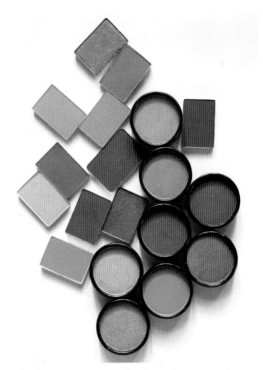

Blushes in a range of colors, from pearl, nude, and dusty pink to orange, coral, and russet.

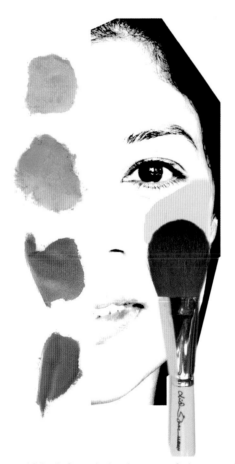

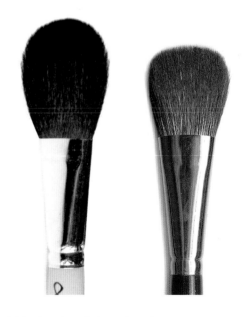

Use mineral blush for a light dusting of shine and color over the cheeks.

A blusher brush (LEFT) and a contouring brush.

applying blush for a visual lift

The brightening that we may need as we age isn't achieved by applying more product, but by changing the type and positioning of those we use to give a lift to our features and enliven our skin. The easiest way to give the face a lift with blush is to blend a touch of soft pink cream blush high on the cheekbone.

As you can see from the photos of Brooke (opposite), adjusting the placement of your blusher even slightly can affect the shape of the face. If you adjust the positioning of your blusher to alter your face shape, be aware of the danger areas shown on page 38 to avoid placing products with problematic color or sheen too near the nose or too far down on the face.

BELOW: As seen here on Lilo, a light touch of cream blush applied high on the cheekbone, just below and slightly behind the outer corners of the eyes, will give the face a visual lift.

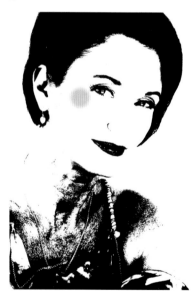

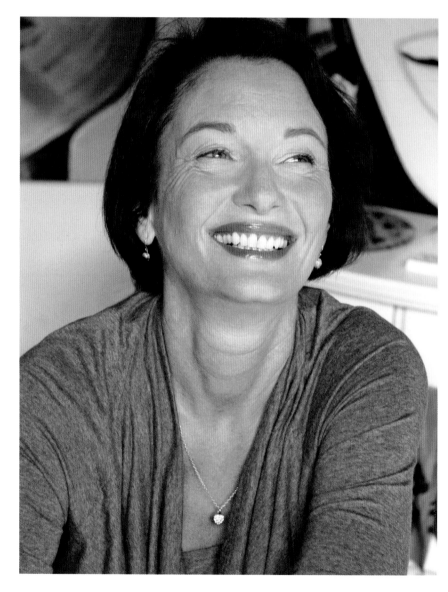

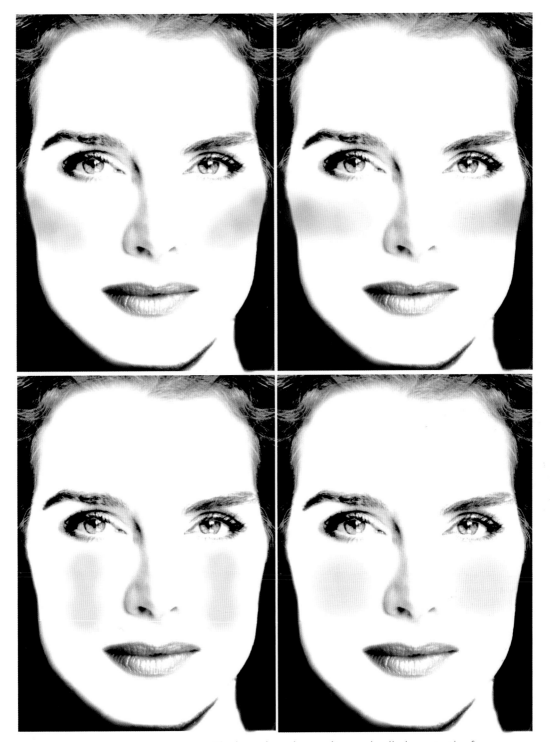

CLOCKWISE FROM TOP LEFT: Blusher placed on a diagonal will elongate the face; blusher placed horizontally will shorten the face; blusher placed vertically will narrow and lengthen the face; blusher placed on the apples of the cheeks will round the face and give a healthy glow.

color for lips

The right lip color and sheen can give any makeup look a beautiful, sophisticated finish.

Lipstick: Matte lipsticks are great for defining lips and achieving a polished look. They tend not to bleed, and applying translucent powder around the lips increases their durability. They can also be applied and rubbed off slightly for a more stained effect. By contrast, cream lipsticks won't last as long.

For those who have trouble keeping lipstick on, long-lasting or indelible types of lipstick that can only be removed with a special product are great and won't bleed, and they can also be used to just stain the lips with color.

Lip gloss and gel: A variety of different types of lip glosses and gels are available, some greasier than others; which one you choose is ultimately a question of personal taste. Lip glosses wear off quickly, while lip gels tend to stay on pretty well.

If you have full lips and want to try strong and bright eye makeup, you may find it easier to use a tinted gloss, like Jan Jaffe (see page 170) and Anna Bayle (page 118, who are wearing black-tinted gloss, which is a simple, elegant way to deepen natural color of the lips.

Lip pencil: These can be used to better define lips, or to gently stain them with color.

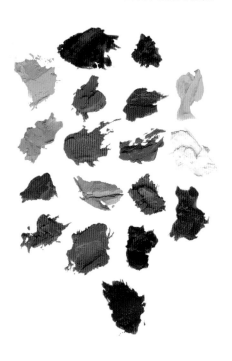

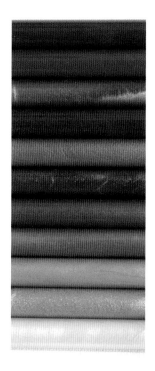

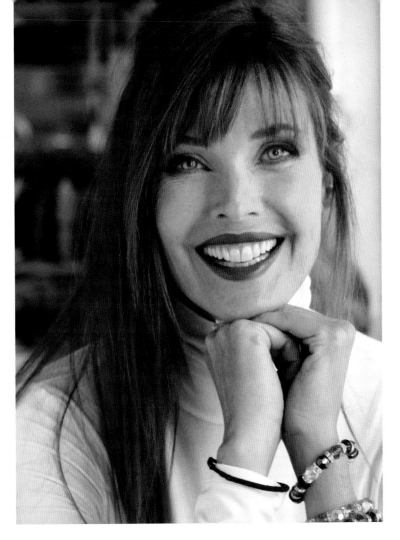

Carol in a daytime look featuring a bright lipcolor balanced with a soft, neutral eye.

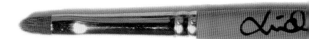

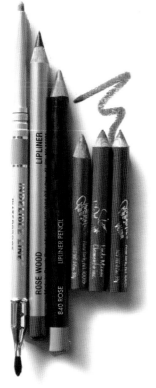

OPPOSITE AND LEFT: Lipsticks in a variety of colors and sheens; lip glosses and lip gels; lip pencils.

ABOVE: A lip brush is a must-have for anyone whose lips need more definition or a fuller appearance.

creating voluptuous lips

To make the lips more voluptuous, imparting softness and enlarging them slightly, define them with a soft beige lip pencil in a slightly deeper color than the natural color of your lips. Go to the very edge of the lighter outline around the lips (a very faint line just slightly beyond the more prominent lip line) so it doesn't look artificial.

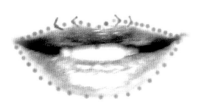

1. Working from the center out, apply the pencil to the lower lip first. Then do the points of the upper lip, starting with the larger side if they're asymmetrical; match the other side to the first by lightly going over the lip edge if necessary.

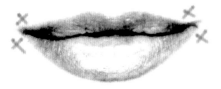

2. Take special care with the corners of the mouth so the lines there aren't too far from the original line.

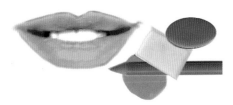

3. Smile; then, using the flat edge of your lip brush, blend the color at the edge of the lips so it's smooth. Take your small powder brush and dab translucent powder around the lip line.

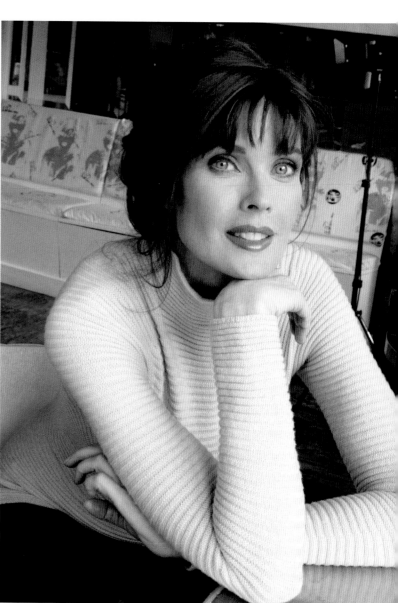

Carol's beautiful lips are made more voluptuous with the right application of lip pencil and color.

correcting asymmetrical lips

If your lips are thin or asymmetrical, you can build them up with lipstick, but it's important to do this carefully, especially when using a strong color, because improperly applied lipstick can actually make lips look thinner and accentuate their asymmetry. This correction is best done with a matte lipstick; if you try using a pencil, the sharper edge may make the lips look too harsh and strongly defined. If you do use a pencil, apply it after you've applied the lipstick, then blend it into the lipstick to give it a softer edge.

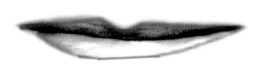

1. Outlining or applying color to asymmetrical lips without correcting their irregularities will only emphasize their unevenness.

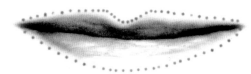

2. With lipstick on your lip brush, outline the upper lip, beginning from the center outward, rounding the points of the bow and edging past the more defined lip edge. For the lower lip, also begin in the center and work outward, noting where the asymmetry is and correcting it.

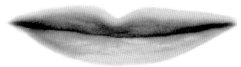

3. Lightly fill in the color, then talk and smile to yourself so that you can see where you might need to further enlarge or even out the edges of the lower lip.

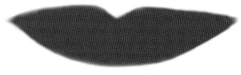

4. With your mouth very relaxed and your lips together, finish filling in with color, correcting the upper lip if you weren't successful the first time.

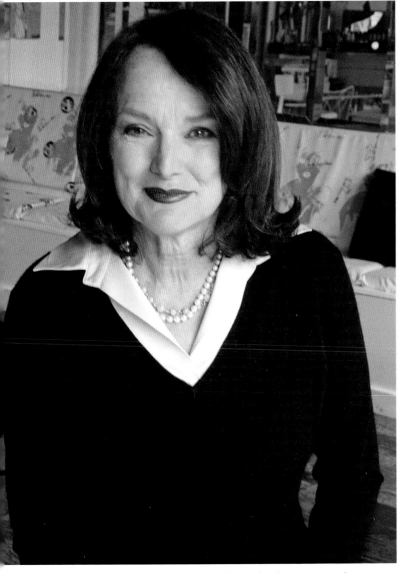

Barbara wearing a matte lipstick applied to correct her irregular lip line. (See pages 138–139 for details on this look.)

playing with color: red lipstick

Having a good-quality red lipstick in your makeup wardrobe is the fastest and easiest way to achieve a pulled-together, elegant look. In fact, you can easily get away with wearing just red lipstick, especially if you have good skin; otherwise, it's best to apply a base and powder first, or at least hide any blemishes with concealer.

The easy way to choose a red is to consider hair color: red with an orange undertone is best for blondes and redheads (think Marilyn Monroe and Annette Bening); for brunettes with pale skin (think Elizabeth Taylor) and darker-skinned women, a blue undertone is most often the best. For myself, a redhead, I feel very comfortable wearing a red lipstick with an orange undertone, but in certain circumstances I like wearing one with a blue undertone, or even a ruby red. I can't just throw those on as I do a bright orange-red, but I can make them look good by adjusting the rest of my makeup.

More than any other lip color, red requires careful, precise application. If you have well-shaped, full lips, then applying the lipstick directly from the tube should work well, but for most women a lip brush is key to ensuring that lip shape is well defined and the color won't accentuate any asymmetry (see page 77). Most lips are asymmetrical, so decide which side you prefer, then match the other side to its shape. Once you've filled in the lower lip, wipe a little color off the corners because too much tends to bring the mouth down.

A rainbow of reds (clockwise from top left): burgundy, bright red with an orange undertone, ruby red, deep burgundy, brick with a rose undertone, brick, and bright red.

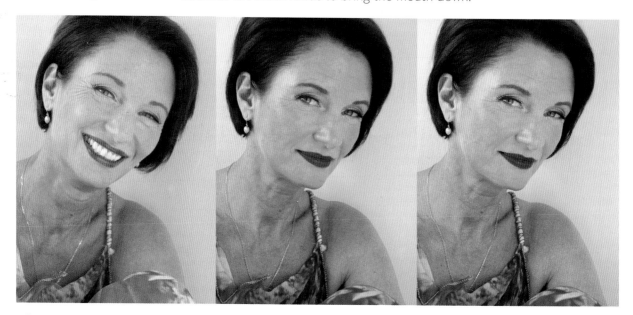

Lilo wearing three different reds (left to right): brick-red, dark violet-red, and bright red.

Keep in mind that a red lipstick may look vivid in the tube, but it may not look as strong when you apply it because it's actually translucent or thin in consistency. When choosing a red, I recommend getting one that's more opaque, because it's easier to tone it down by blotting or rubbing lightly than it is to strengthen a translucent one, unless you apply a heavy pencil of the same color underneath it.

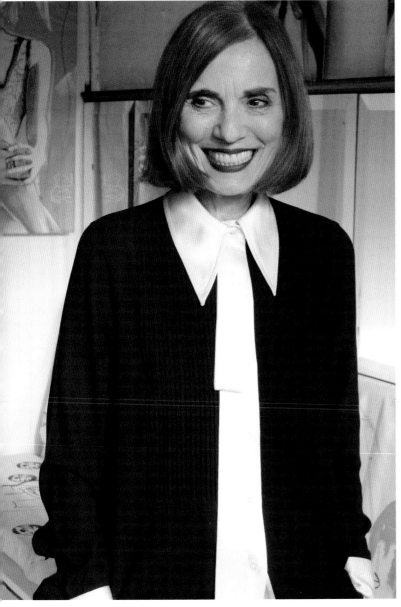

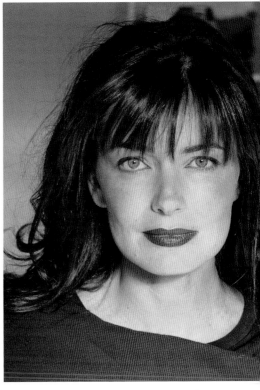

LEFT: Felicia Milewicz, beauty director of *Glamour* magazine, was told by cosmetics industry pioneer Estée Lauder that she should always wear red, which both accentuates her pale skin and conveys her vibrant, fun-loving personality.
ABOVE: Paulina Porizkova in bright red lipstick. (For more on this look, see pages 134–135.)

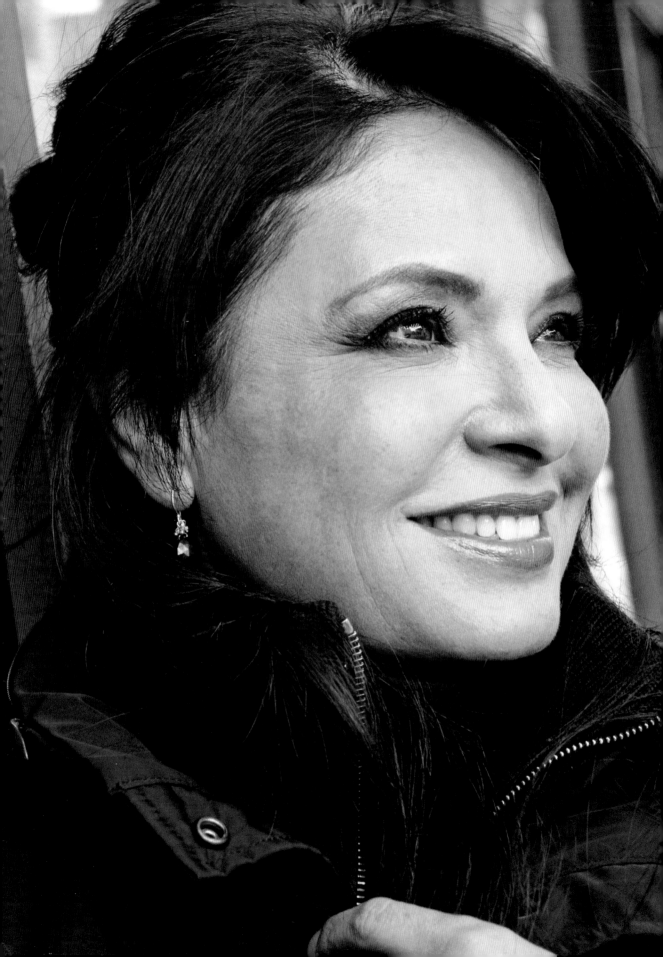

4. subtle looks

Subtle color is makeup for every day that gives your appearance and spirit a gentle lift. The looks in this chapter range from delicate touches of brown to lightly accentuate fading brows and lashes to golds and pinks that soften strong features and enhance a natural elegance.

Doris in a simple look for everyday that enhances her natural beauty. (For more about Doris, see page 98–101.)

strengthening
fading features

Silko Coelenbier 60s

Silko is an artist from the Camargue area in Provence, France, who creates her art from antique French textiles. She spends a lot of time outdoors, so she wanted a makeup that would freshen and brighten her appearance but that she could feel comfortable wearing every day, even while horseback riding.

Because I want to show the subtle effects of a gel base, I've included a "before" photo of Silko without makeup. I first used a warm medium shade of gel base to even out the skin and make it more matte. I then applied a medium shade of concealer to the inner corners of her eyes. When applying blush, I focused on Silko's cheekbones and took care to avoid the apples of her cheeks, where she already had some redness.

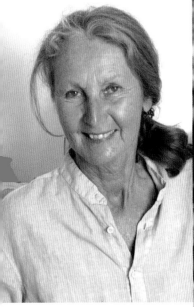

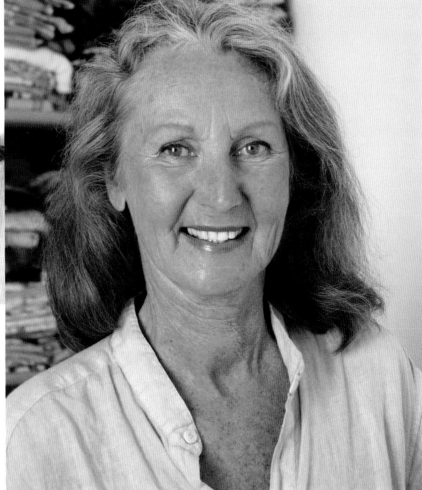

Silko as she spends her days in her studio (ABOVE) and as she looks after a light application of a gel base and a little concealer, along with simple makeup in neutral colors (see opposite for details).

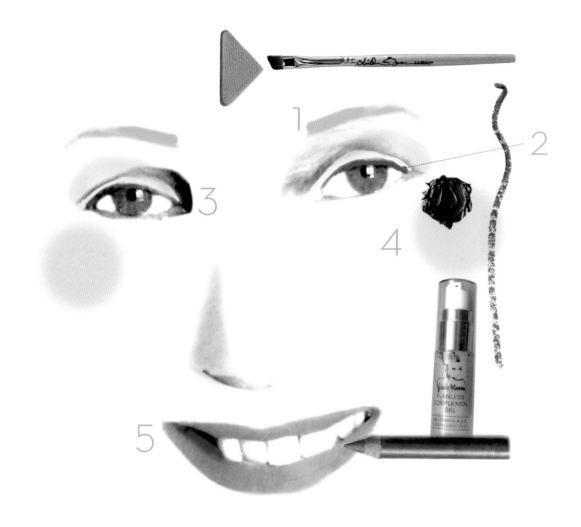

the "no makeup" makeup

1 **Eyebrows:** To thicken and accentuate virtually nonexistent brows, use the angled brow brush to apply a semipearl beige mushroom eye shadow or eyebrow powder.

2 **Eye liner:** Work a little gray pencil into the base of the upper lashes to give them definition but without making a hard line.

3 **Eye shadow/mascara:** Using the small eye shadow brush, blend the semipearl beige mushroom shade used on the brows from the base of the upper eyelashes to just past the crease. Apply black or brown mascara to the upper lashes.

4 **Blush:** Dot a touch of reddish-brown cream blush on the cheekbone, blending it high and away from the apples of the cheeks as needed to avoid emphasizing redness.

5 **Lip color:** To deepen and define pale lips, use a lip pencil in a natural pink. Finish with clear gloss.

lightening and updating
a retro look

Bibi Lencek 50s

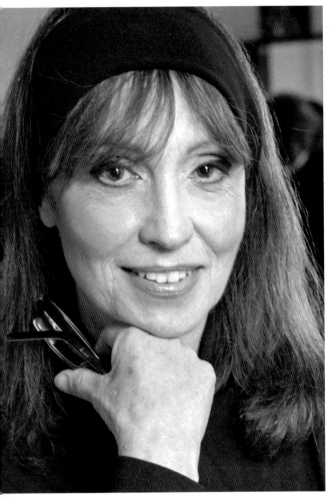

Bibi, a fine artist and art teacher, enjoys transforming and improving her looks with makeup. For her, makeup is fun and gives her self-confidence. For her everyday makeup, Bibi likes the focus to be on her eyes. Her lashes and brows are light and her eyes quite recessed, so she feels they disappear unless she accentuates them. She also wears moisturizer, concealer, blush, and eye liner, and applies lipstick if she has time.

Bibi has always liked a heavily lined 1960s-style eye and needed reassurance that continuing this practice wouldn't age her. We decided to stick with her look and take the eye liner to the next level for that retro look she admires. Thanks to her youthful style, it doesn't look old-fashioned on her but rather timely and fresh. The goal for this look is to give the face and eyes a lift by starting with a thin line in the center of the lid, thickening it gradually as it moves toward the outer lid. Also, it's important to give the skin adequate but not heavy coverage by applying a thin layer of cream base as near as possible to the natural skin tone, and using very little blush and a soft lip color. Applying too heavy or dark a base, lip color, or bronzer with this eye makeup would create an aging heaviness.

We first evened out Bibi's skin tone using a mixture of two very light shades of cream base, blending them with a damp sponge, then applied a light cream concealer underneath and to the inner and outer corners of her eyes with a small brush. For the eye makeup, we used a matte white shadow over the entire eyelid, then a matte dark brown shadow in the crease, making sure it didn't go into the deep part near Bibi's nose, and blended it slightly over the bone. The liner used was a creamy ebony black pencil. Bibi's lashes are very light, so we made sure to get into the very base of the lashes with the pencil to strengthen them.

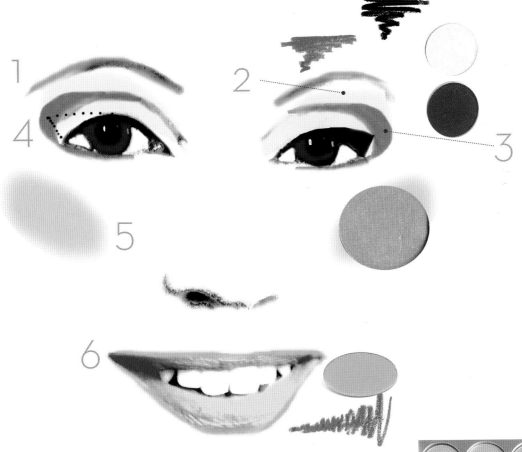

retro with a modern twist

1 **Eyebrows:** Gently go over the brows with a blond pencil.

2 **Eye shadow/highlight:** Apply a matte white shadow over the entire eyelid to lighten the eye socket.

3 **Eye shadow/shading:** Using your small eye shadow brush, blend a dark brown matte shadow into the crease, making sure it doesn't go into the deepest-set area, near the nose. Blend the color slightly over the bone and at the base of the lower lashes.

4 **Eye liner/mascara:** Use a creamy ebony black eye pencil to thoroughly color the very base of the upper lashes, but don't apply it all the way to the outer end of the eye. Then make a dot where you would like the eye liner to end (about at the crease). Draw a line upward from the end of the penciling to the dot; then draw a line from where the rim of the eye starts descending to the end of this short upward line. If your eyelashes are very sparse and you've correctly penciled in the base of the lashes, you won't need mascara.

5 **Blush:** Apply just a hint of a very soft blush.

6 **Lip color:** Apply a nude lip color, then line the lips with a beige pencil, blending the liner into the lip color so it isn't too strong.

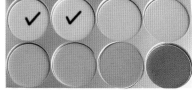

The colors of cream base I used on Bibi.

BEAUTY CHALLENGE:
deep-set eyes

We used concealer to lighten up the inner corners of Bibi's eyes, next to the nose where they're the most sunken, and in the crease under her eyes to give their outer corners a lift before applying the eye liner. When applying the concealer, we took care to avoid using it in the areas that had the most smile lines and used matte eye shadows so as not to emphasize those same lines.

minimal chic
Kikan Massara 60s

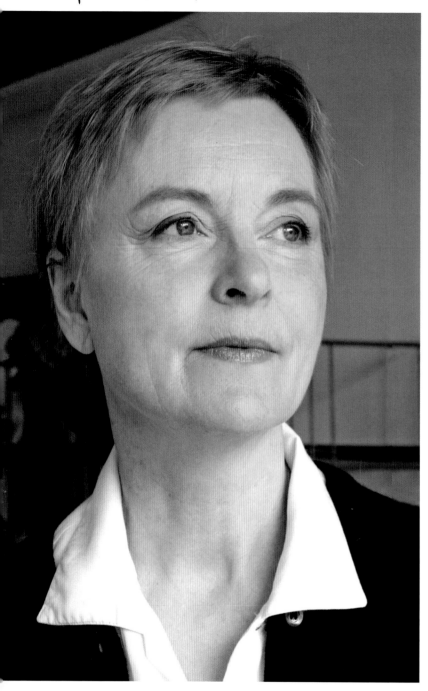

Kikan and I worked together in Paris at the end of the 1970s and during the early '80s, when she was modeling for all the designers every year. This gave us a lot of time to develop a friendship, and we remain friends today. Now living in Paris, Kikan is a psychotherapist, life coach, and writer who's also working on some very exciting self-help projects.

I started this look by evening out Kikan's skin tone with a light shade of liquid base, then applied a light beige cream concealer to the inner corners of her eyes, her eyelids, and very lightly under her eyes. I finished her skin with a very light application of translucent powder, but only around her nose, chin, and forehead. Kikan has very fair brows and short, rather thin and straight upper lashes, and since mascara alone is rarely enough to make these kinds of lashes look thicker, even when it's generously applied, I rubbed a soft gray eyeliner pencil into their base to give them subtle strength, but without a defined line.

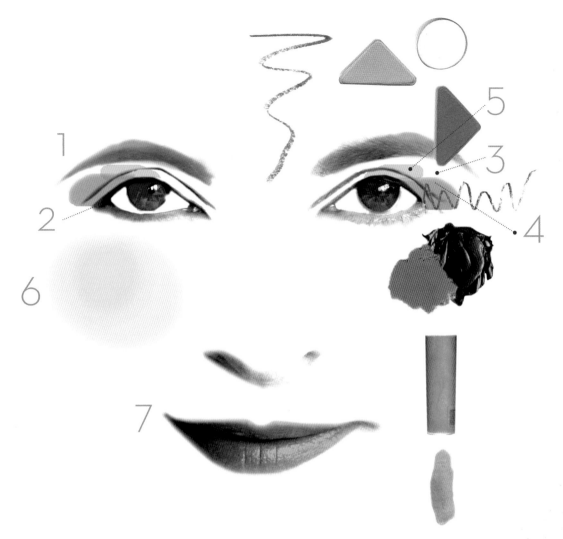

simple makeup for every day

1 **Eyebrows:** Use a blond eyebrow pencil to fill in sparse areas. Lightly rub the pencil over the brow hairs to strengthen them visually, then use it to define the brows' arches and length.

2 **Lashes:** Dot gray pencil into the base of the upper lashes, then soften it with a mini-eye shadow brush.

3 **Eye shadow/highlight:** Apply a matte white over the entire lid.

4 **Eye shadow/deep tone:** Use a small eye shadow brush to press a touch of a light warm brown matte shadow onto the outer upper corners of the eyes, then blend it upward and outward.

5 **Eye shadow/accent:** Apply a soft matte gray-green onto the center of the eyelid where the white and brown meet, then lightly blend it into both.

6 **Blush:** Use your fingertips to blend a mixture of warm red-brown and light pink cream blushes onto the apples of the cheeks.

7 **Lip color:** Soften the lips with a slightly pearlescent pink lipgloss.

timeless femininity
Brooke Shields 40s

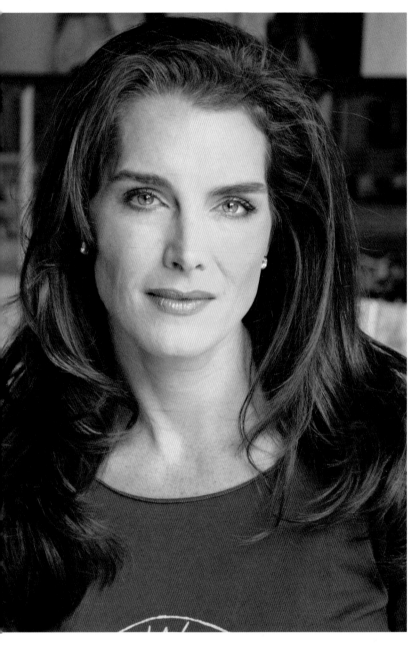

I worked with Brooke many times in the late 1980s and early 1990s but hadn't had the opportunity to make her up for quite some time since then, so it was wonderful to be able to do so for this book. She has perfect features: almond-shaped eyes, great cheekbones, beautifully shaped lips, and of course those memorable eyebrows, which are so much a part of her beauty.

I started Brooke's first makeup look with a thin layer of lightweight, water-based liquid base, then used a concealer brush to apply a light-colored concealer to the inside upper corners of and below the eyes, finishing with a very light dusting of translucent powder over the face. For her first look, I accentuated her features with soft color and her eyes with a light touch of silver shadow. After delicately defining her almond-shaped eyes by applying a very soft beige shadow to the crease and under the eye, I brought out the upper lashes with a light silver shadow at their base. Then I added a touch of silver to the inner corner of the lower rim of the eyes. Next I applied a soft dusty pink powder blusher from the cheekbone onto the apples of the cheeks. I finished the makeup with a light pink lip gloss and a beige lip pencil.

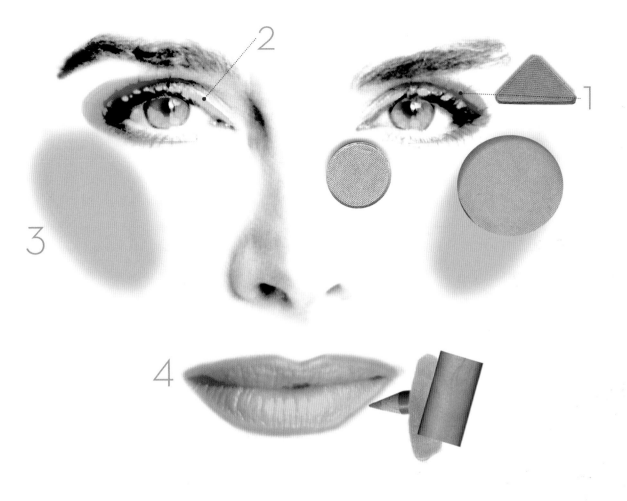

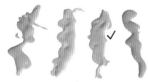

The color of liquid base I used on Brooke.

muted shimmer

1 **Eye shadow/midtone:** Using a small eye shadow brush, blend a mushroom-colored semipearl shadow into the crease and over the brow bone in the outer two-thirds of the eye.

2 **Eye shadow/highlight:** Apply silver eye shadow to the base of the upper lashes.

3 **Blush:** Use a blusher brush to apply a dusty pink powder blush to the cheekbone, and then blend it downward, onto the apples of the cheeks.

4 **Lip color:** Apply a light pink lip gloss, followed by a beige lip pencil.

BEAUTY CHALLENGE: strong brows

With the combination of a strong brow and an almond-shaped eye, it's both easier and more flattering to keep eye makeup soft and simple because there's limited space between the brow and the eye, giving you less room to play with color.

delicate color

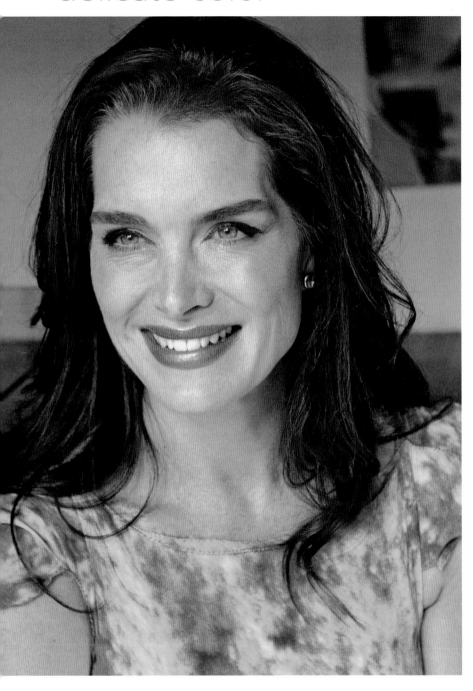

For Brooke's second, more glamorous look, rather than a fashion statement I wanted something more timeless, a makeup that accentuates femininity.

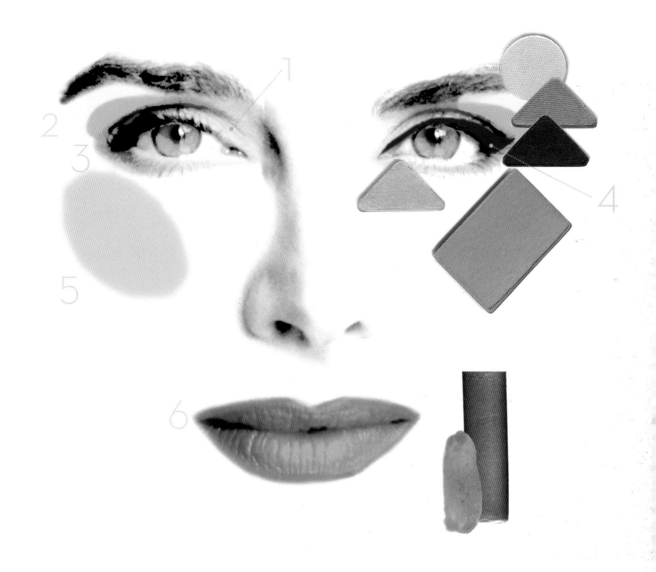

1 **Eye liner/highlight:** Blend iridescent pale blue around the eye at the base of the upper and lower lashes.

2 **Eye shadow/highlight:** Apply a matte bone color over the brow bone, under the eyebrow.

3 **Eye shadow/midtone:** Blend semipearl mushroom shadow in the crease of the eye.

4 **Eye liner/accents:** Apply black cake liner at the base of the upper lashes, making the line thicker toward the outer corners of the eyes. Apply white pencil inside the rims of the lower lids.

5 **Blush:** Blend coral powder blush in from the cheekbone to the apples of the cheeks.

6 **Lip color:** Start with a pink lip color that matches the natural color of the lips, then enhance with a deep pink lip gloss. If desired, add a touch of white pearl shimmer.

looking good on camera

Dana Roc 40's

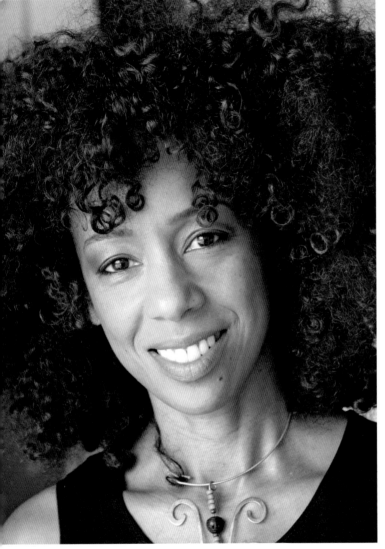

Dana has been a client of mine for many years. As an actress, motivational speaker, and founder of *Dana Delivered!*, an e-zine filled with interesting stories and fun tidbits, it's important that she look good on camera.

Dana has very fine skin but feels that it doesn't photograph as well as it looks in real life. She wears a tinted moisturizer, a touch of color on the eyes, and a pale pink lip color daily, so we did some experimenting with a couple of different bases to find something suitable for her camera work. This was tricky because there are so many different lighting possibilities on a shoot.

We decided that a simple, modern makeup with a touch of color was the best way to go with Dana. However, this type of makeup has a tendency to disappear under strong lights in a studio, or if you're being photographed in a group, such as at a wedding (where you may not be ideally lit because you're not the focus of the photo). In this type of situation it's important that you pay special attention to the finish of your skin, the evening out of your skin tone, and the blending of your colors. For this look of Dana's I used a mixture of two cream bases and a little concealer. If your skin is darker like Dana's, finish your base makeup by applying translucent powder with a small powder brush around the nostrils, to the chin, and to the center of the forehead, then use a darker powder with more pigment and coverage to matte the apples of the cheeks, which often attract too much light on darker skin.

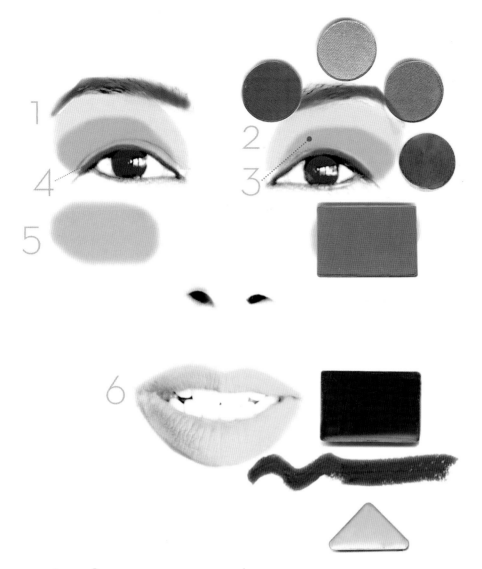

ready for your closeup

1 **Eyebrows:** Define brows with a little dark brown powder applied with the angled brow brush.

2 **Eye shadow/highlight:** Apply a soft, slightly iridescent pinky beige over the brow bone with a large eye shadow brush.

3 **Eye shadow/midtone:** Apply a slightly iridescent burgundy to the lid and in the crease of the eye.

4 **Eye liner:** Use bright blue gel eye liner to accentuate eye shape and enhance (or contrast with) skin tone.

5 **Blush:** Apply a matte russet blush. (Dana has a long, narrow face, so I applied it horizontally to round it out.)

6 **Lip color:** A soft, pale '60s-style pinky nude (shown here), black gloss, or a bright red (see page 78) both work beautifully with this look. To give the red a very matte look, press on a red powder eye shadow over the lipstick.

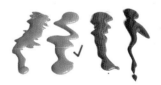

The colors of liquid and cream base I used on Dana.

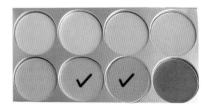

subtle yet sexy

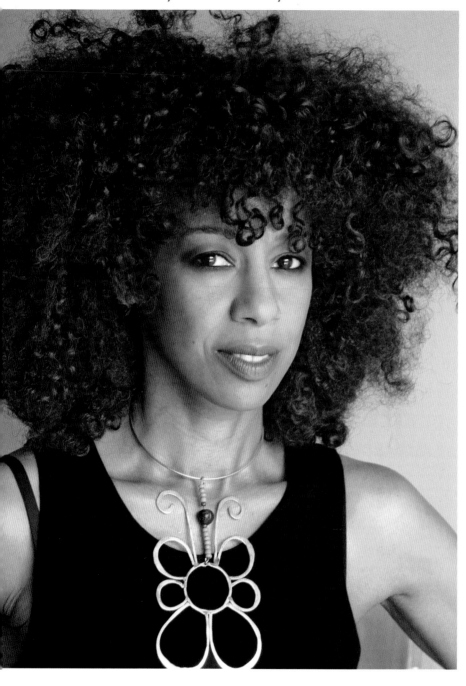

For this look, Dana wanted to experiment with a smoky eye (see page 64). Like a classic handbag, the smoky eye will never go out of style, but I didn't think it would convey Dana's original and spontaneous personality, especially on camera. So I designed a fresh look with a glamorous touch that still maintains Dana's individuality. I gave her eyes a slight smoky strength with matte neutrals, using them in the crease and on her browbone, kept the lips natural with a soft pink, and combined two very soft matte blush colors for the cheeks.

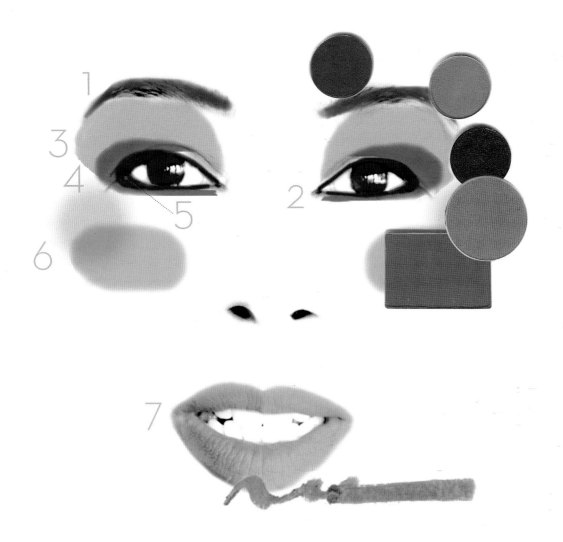

1 **Eyebrows:** Lightly powder the brows with dark brown shadow using the angled brow brush.

2 **Eye liner:** Apply black eye pencil to the inner rim of the lower lashes and at the very base of the upper and lower lashes, then blend with a mini-eye shadow brush.

3 **Eye shadow/highlight:** Brush a matte taupe over the entire eyelid.

4 **Eye shadow/midtone:** Use a mini-eye shadow brush to blend a dark brown matte shadow into the crease of the eye and beneath the eyes at the base of the lower lashes.

5 **Eye shadow/deep tone:** Press a black shadow into the penciling around the eye and blend it into the edges of the dark brown shadow.

6 **Blush:** Apply a matte russet blush horizontally across the apples of the cheeks, then add a touch of bright pink powder blush to the cheekbone.

7 **Lip color:** Use a soft matte pink lipstick.

all-american woman

Kim Alexis 40s

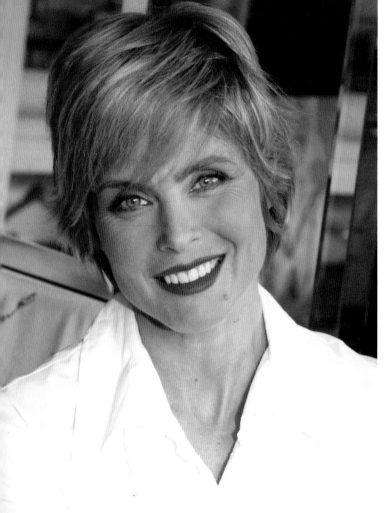

Kim, a spokesperson and model, has a jeans clothing line called "Curve Appeal." She's very upbeat and lives a healthy lifestyle, so both her body and her face are in great shape. With her distinctive cheekbones and clear blue eyes, she's hardly changed since I last worked with her more than ten years ago.

Because Kim has a slight tan, I decided to warm and slightly deepen her complexion. She's the ideal candidate for tinted moisturizers for everyday use, but I decided to go with a little more coverage for these photos, a polished look that also works well for special events. I mixed two warm bases—one quite yellow and the other more red—then blended and applied them lightly using a damp sponge so they were almost imperceptible. I applied concealer to the inner corners of the eyes and sparingly to the outer corners and under the eyes. I then lightly used translucent powder only on the center of the face, around the nostrils and chin, and in the inner corners of her eyes. After applying eyes, lips, and blush, I finished the entire face with a light dusting of bronzing powder.

This warm, harmonious makeup application is traditionally used to accentuate cool blue eyes. The warmth of all the peachy browns and gold contrasts with and emphasizes their color. Keep lips russet during the day for softness, then use a brighter brick-colored lipstick to transition to an evening look.

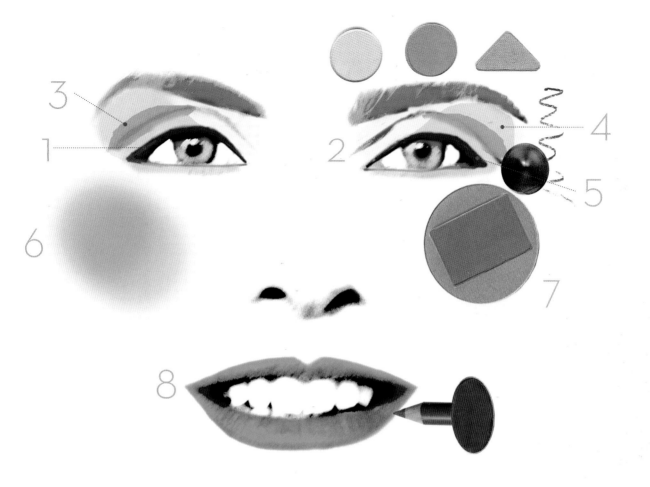

accentuating blue eyes

1 **Eye liner:** Using brown pencil liner, pencil the base of the upper lashes a third of the way in from the outer corners of the eyes.

2 **Eye shadow/highlight:** Blend in a matte peachy-white at the inner corners of the eyes.

3 **Eye shadow/midtone:** Blend a matte beige into the crease of the eye and press it onto the brown pencil line at the base of the lashes.

4 **Eye shadow/accent:** Blend gold over the matte shading, past the crease of the eye and toward the brow; apply a little under the eyes.

5 **Eye liner/mascara:** Apply a thin line of brown gel liner to the base of the upper lashes, thickening it slightly at the outer corners of the eyes. Apply black mascara to both the upper and the lower lashes.

6 **Blush:** Blend a little matte russet blush onto the cheekbones and the apples of the cheeks.

7 **Bronzing powder:** Lightly brush bronzer over the blush and around the face.

8 **Lip color:** Apply a brick lip color, then define the lips with a lip pencil in the same shade.

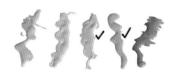

The colors of liquid base I used on Kim.

day into evening
Doris Lozada 50s

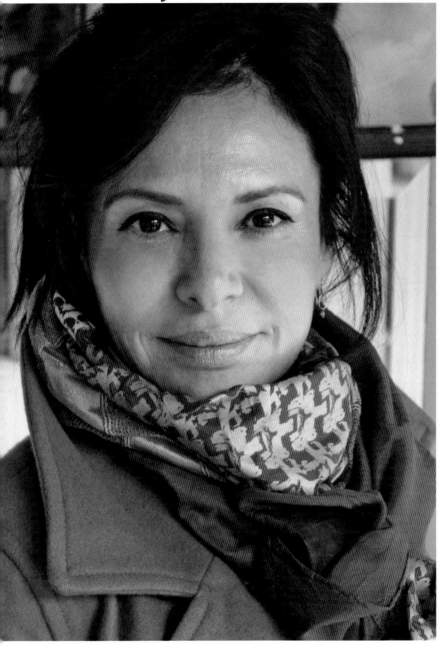

Doris is the owner of a contracting and renovation company she started twenty years ago, when there were virtually no women in the field. At that time she believed that makeup would draw too much attention on construction sites, so she didn't wear any. About four years ago, however, she came to see me. After being very fearful and worried about looking too made-up, she's become ever bolder and has since come to love wearing makeup, which she has on all the time. According to Doris, "Construction is a man's world, and by wearing makeup I found a way to maintain my femininity."

For every day, Doris applies a deep, rich golden yellow liquid base to warm up her skin tone, then blends some concealer around her eyes. She also wears a dark brown gel eye liner and mascara and slightly thickens her eyebrows with pencils. Completing the look is a nude lip color over black gloss and an orange blush that brightens her cheeks. After wearing only the black lip gloss for a few years, she now has a "wardrobe" of lip colors she likes to choose from.

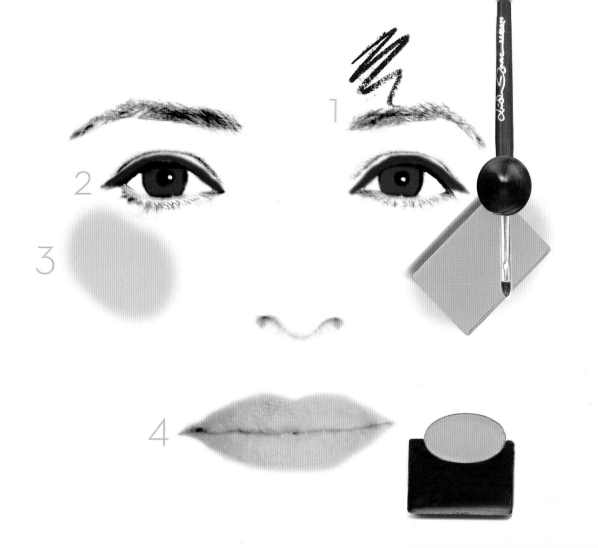

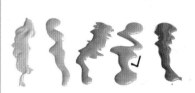

day-to-day

1 **Eyebrows:** Thicken the brows slightly with a dark brown eyebrow pencil.

2 **Eye liner/mascara:** Line the base of the upper lashes with a thin line of brown gel eye liner. Apply black mascara.

3 **Blush:** Blend an orange powder blush on the apples of the cheeks.

4 **Lip color:** Apply a nude lipstick over black gloss.

BEAUTY CHALLENGE:
making olive skin glow

The choice of the base was most important here because this element is primarily what makes someone feel made-up, especially women like Doris who have olive skin. The base I chose was a lightweight, deep warm yellow that blended with her natural olive tone, brightening it without looking heavy or masklike.

evening transformation

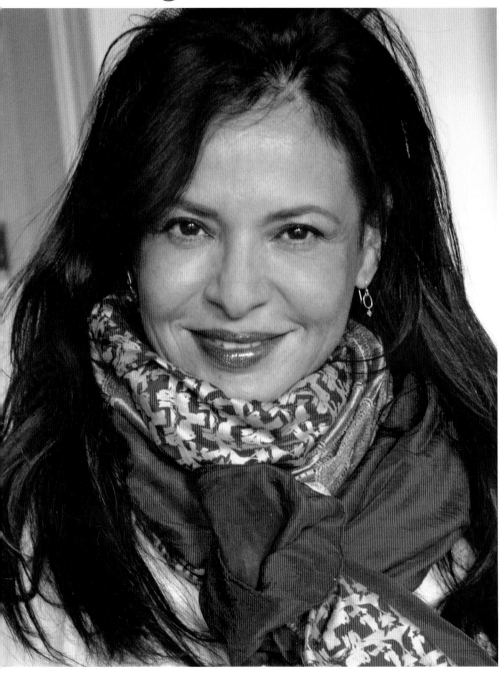

For this look, Doris is wearing essentially the same liquid base and concealer as described on page 98, but we added more coverage by blending two colors of cream base. We also chose slightly stronger colors for the eyes and lips, which makes it appropriate as a transitional look from a day at work to a fun night out.

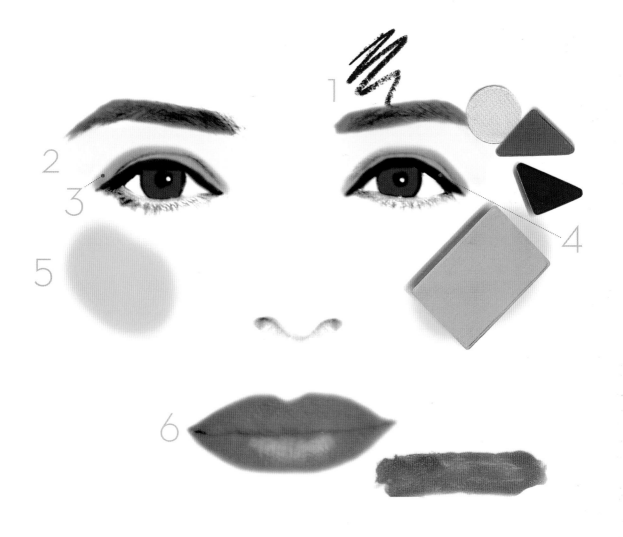

1 **Eyebrows:** Fill in and thicken brows more heavily with a dark brown pencil.

2 **Eye shadow/highlight:** Apply a pale beige eye shadow with a slight sheen under the eyebrows.

3 **Eye shadow/midtone:** Apply a warm russet shadow to the crease of the eye and a little above it.

4 **Eye liner/mascara:** Strengthen the brown eye liner gel by applying a thin line of black cake eye liner over it. Add two more coats of black mascara.

5 **Blush:** Blend orange powder on the apples of the cheeks.

6 **Lip color:** Apply a lip gel in a deep berry over a paler lipstick.

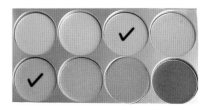

The two colors of cream base I used for this look.

fresh-faced and energized

Mimi Quillin 50s

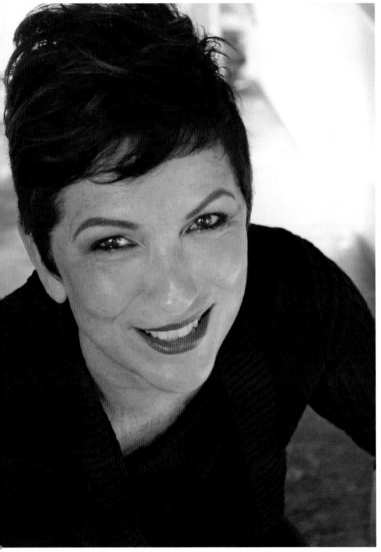

Mimi is a friendly and enthusiastic actress, dancer, and Pilates teacher. She was introduced to makeup while she was an actress in New York City, and other actresses and theater professionals would share tips and tricks with one another. When Mimi is working at her Pilates practice, she makes sure to wear a little lipstick, pencils in her eyebrows, and applies kohl inside the inner rim of her lower lashes. She believes that makeup is important for making her feel confident about her appearance, and can even motivate her to work out because it's an easy way to feel better about your appearance that can inspire you to improve yourself in other ways, such as by taking care of your health. "I feel better when I look in the mirror," she admits, "and I don't look awful." Some of her beauty secrets? Mimi swears by drinking stinging nettle-infusion tea for her skin as well as lots of water. She uses yoga balls to erase facial lines.

As Mimi has gotten older, she's learned to make necessary changes in her makeup routine. Some of these include wearing darker eyebrow makeup and lip color. She regularly wears base, blush, eye shadow, mascara, eye liner, and lipstick, and often changes her makeup routine from day to day, using lighter makeup during the summer. Mimi feels it's necessary to use a little bit more makeup as she ages because the skin tends to lose some of its pigment over the years.

For this look, I very finely applied a thin layer of a warm-colored liquid base to her face.

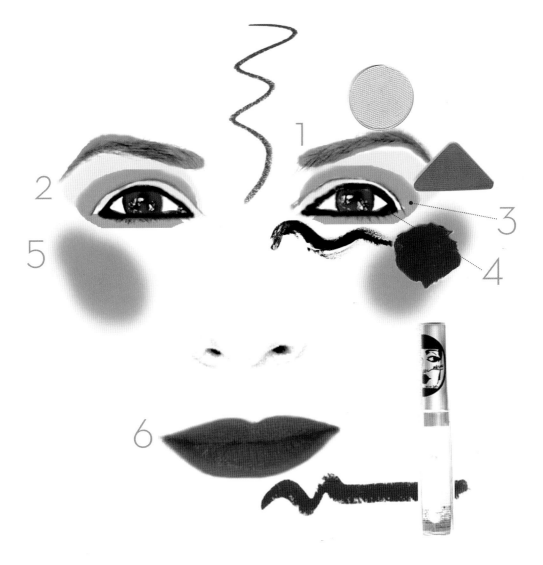

subtle sophistication

1 **Eyebrows:** Shape and thicken the eyebrows with a brunette eyebrow pencil.

2 **Eye shadow/highlight:** Blend a soft matte pale pink over the entire eyelid using a large eye shadow brush.

3 **Eye shadow/midtone:** Using your mini-eye shadow brush, blend a matte yellow brown color into the crease of the eye and under the lower lashes at their base, layering it to make it quite heavy.

4 **Eye liner:** Follow the inner rim of the lower lashes with a black eye liner pencil. Use the same pencil to smudge a little color around the eyes.

5 **Blush:** Blend a reddish brown cream blush down from the cheekbones onto the apples of the cheeks.

6 **Lip color:** Apply a deep red lipstick with a lip brush.

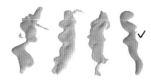

The color of liquid base I chose for Mimi.

modern and matte
Susanna *Midnight 40s*

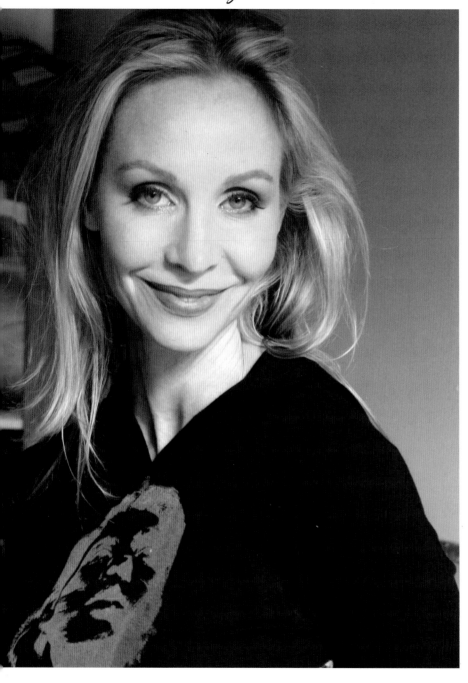

Susanna, a producer and a member of The Actors Studio, appears in my first book, *Makeup: The Art of Beauty*, so I was thrilled that she visited New York from Los Angeles and was able to participate while I was shooting the looks for this book.

For Susanna's base, I used a pale liquid foundation and a very light cream concealer. Her eyes are deep in the inner corners, so I paid a lot of attention to lightening up those areas. Matte gray and gray-green accentuate her green eyes beautifully for a lovely everyday look.

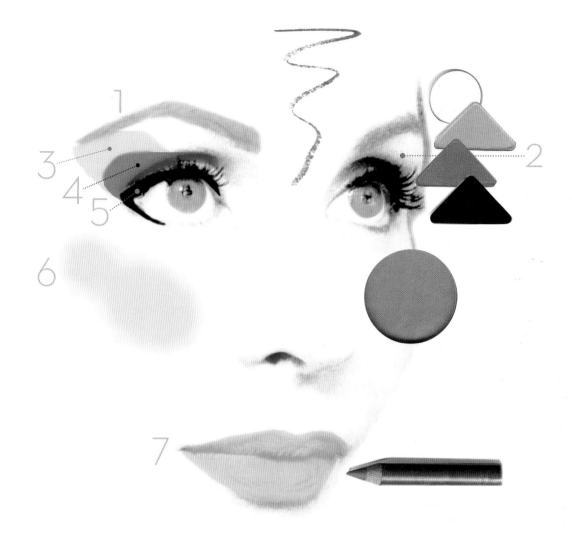

timeless with a touch of color

1 **Eyebrows:** Use a blond pencil to strengthen and define the brows.

2 **Eye shadow/highlight:** Apply a matte white over the entire eyelid with a large eye shadow brush.

3 **Eye shadow/midtone:** With a small eye shadow brush, blend a light matte gray-green from the base of the lashes at the outer area of the eye, tapering off toward the end of the brow.

4 **Eye shadow/deep tone:** Using a mini-eye shadow brush, blend a matte gray into the crease and over the browbone into the gray-green.

5 **Eye liner/mascara:** With a liner brush, blend wet black cake eyeliner into the base of the lashes, starting at the outer corner, then tapering off into the inner corner. Apply black mascara.

6 **Blush:** Blend a soft muted pink down onto the cheekbones on a diagonal.

7 **Lip color:** Stain and define the lips by rubbing them with a subdued pink lip pencil.

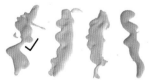

The color of liquid base I used on Susanna.

simple elegance
Claudja Bicalho 50s

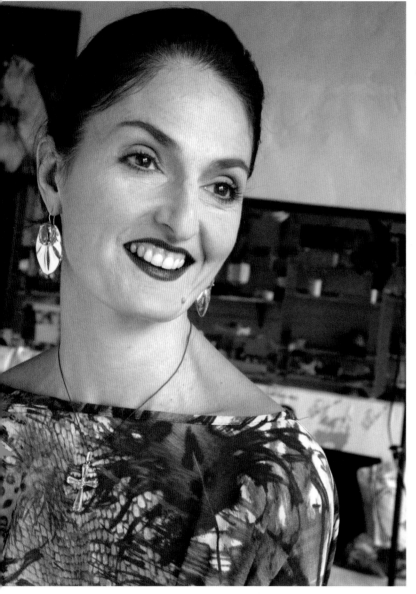

I've known Claudja since she was a model in the late 1980s, and now she designs both jewelry and clothing. She has strong features, great bone structure, and looks great without makeup. Her unusual beauty inspired me to be very creative with her makeup when she was younger, but I was never really happy with what I did. So this time my challenge was to gently accentuate her strong features with a subtle makeup look, which I realized would complement them in the most beautiful way.

Because Claudja has big eyes and really long eyelashes, her main everyday makeup is mascara. Her eyelids are expansive and smooth, so she would look great wearing a dusting of any soft iridescent color over the lid (especially violet or light green). However, because I was planning on using a strong lip color, I opted for an elegant combination of a soft light matte rose combined with a semimatte gold next to the eye (to accentuate the gold in her eyes) and finished with lots of mascara.

For Claudja's skin, I applied a cream base very lightly, then applied concealer under her eyes and in their inner corners, as well as on the brown mark on her cheek. To finish, I pressed the translucent powder onto her forehead, nose, and chin, then dusted it lightly over the rest of the face.

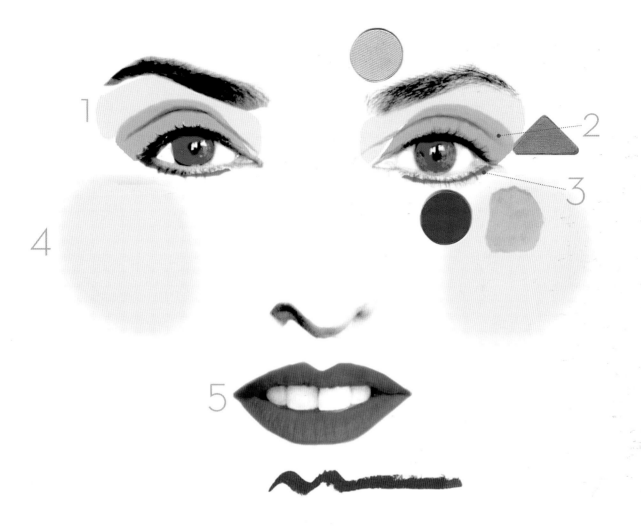

flattering strong features

1. **Eye shadow/highlight:** Dust on a soft matte pink shadow with the large eye shadow brush in the inner corner of the eyes and over the brow bone.

2. **Eye shadow/midtone:** Use the smaller eye shadow brush to blend in gold eye shadow from the base of the lashes to just above the crease of the eye.

3. **Eye shadow/accent:** With the mini-eye shadow brush, press a little matte dark brown shadow into the very base of the lower lashes. Apply black mascara heavily to both the upper and lower lashes.

4. **Blush:** Dust a very pale mineral blush over the cheeks to give them a little sheen.

5. **Lip color:** Define the lips with a pink or reddish pencil, overlapping the edges slightly, then apply a soft deep red. Blot to soften.

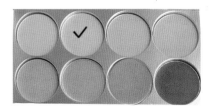

The color of cream base I used on Claudja.

enhancing natural beauty

Gunilla Lindblad 60s

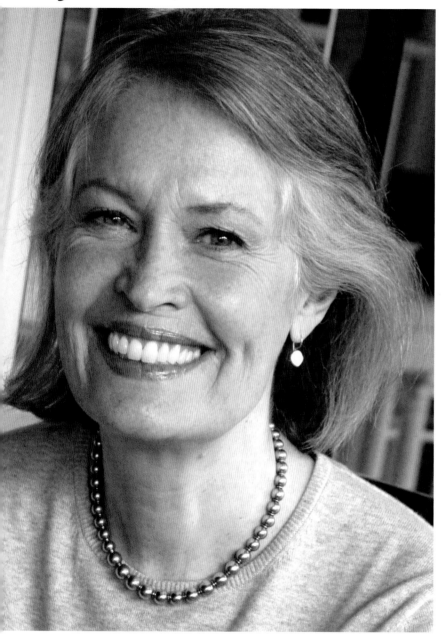

A timeless beauty, Swedish model Gunilla was already at the top of her field when I met her in Paris in the 1970s. Her first job in New York was a twenty-page spread for *Vogue*. Despite her fame, she was often expected to do her own hair and makeup. *Vogue*'s then editor-in-chief, Diana Vreeland, told her, "Do your makeup to match your clothing. If you're wearing violet, do violet makeup." With Gunilla's gray hair (and the sweater she was wearing that day), I felt that gray and taupe were the subtle colors that most discreetly flattered her classic beauty. For women with gray hair, it's important to blend a little gray shadow into their brows after defining them with a slightly darker pencil.

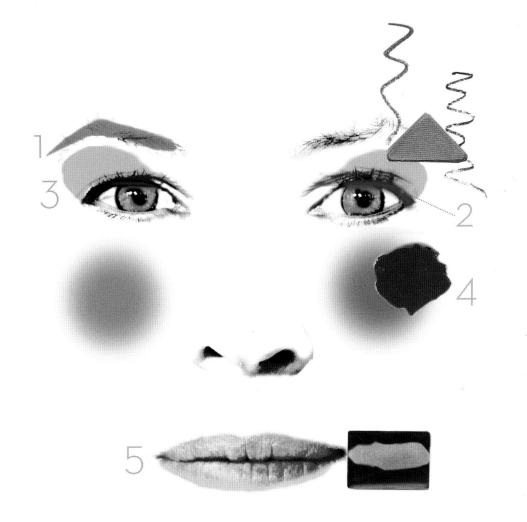

a new classic

1 **Eyebrows:** Use a blond eyebrow pencil to lightly define and fill in the brows.

2 **Eye liner:** Rub a gray pencil into the very base of the upper lashes.

3 **Eye shadow:** Apply a soft beige semipearl shadow from the base of the lashes outward, past the crease of the eye.

4 **Blush:** Blend a deep warm shade of cream blush onto the apples of the cheeks and spread outward.

5 **Lip color:** Apply a black tinted gloss with a soft pink gloss over it.

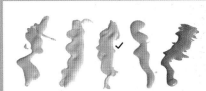

BEAUTY CHALLENGE:
gently warming pale skin

For the base makeup for this look, I used a dot of a liquid base in a slightly deeper shade than Gunilla's skin mixed with moisturizer, blending them well with my fingertips before applying them. The goal was to give Gunilla's skin a bit of warmth while avoiding a "made up" appearance.

fresh and elegant

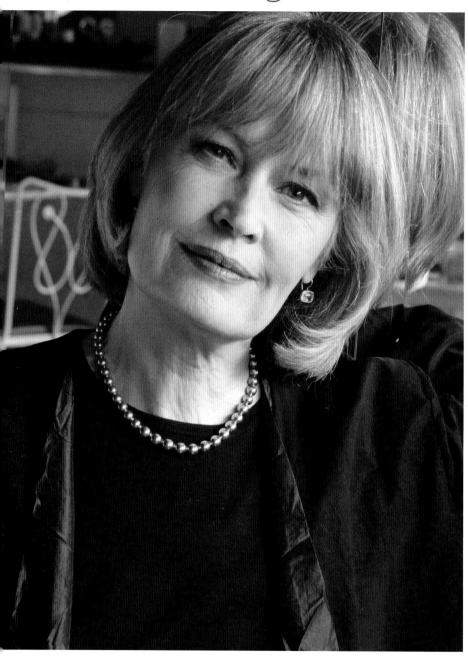

For this makeup, which is a more refined evening look, I started by applying a liquid base that was as close as possible to Gunilla's actual skin tone (a bit lighter than the base used in the New Classic look), then added a little concealer to her eyelids and under the eyes before dusting the entire face lightly with translucent powder. The makeup for the brows is the same, but the placement of the blush is slightly different, a bit higher on the cheekbones.

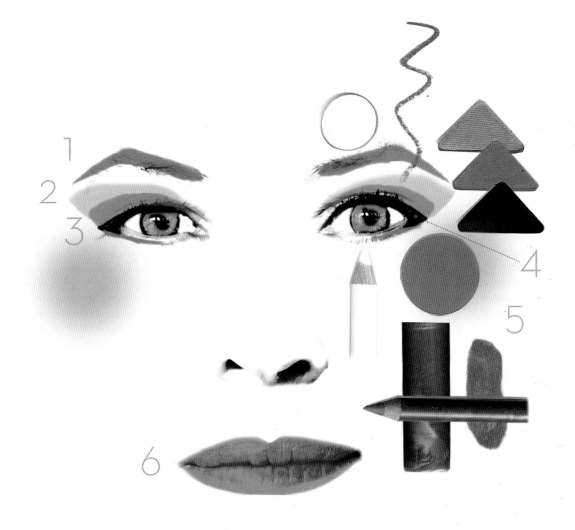

1 **Eyebrows:** Use a blond eyebrow pencil to lightly fill in and define the brows, then apply some gray powder with the angled brow brush.

2 **Eye shadow/highlight:** Blend a soft taupe shadow from the base of the lashes outward, past the fold of the eye and toward the brow. This layer creates a base for the other colors to blend into. Apply white pencil to the inner rim at the lower lashes.

3 **Eye shadow/midtone:** Blend matte gray eye shadow from the base of the lashes over the taupe color to just past the fold, pressing the color into the base of the lashes to make it heavier there. Apply a little under the eye, at the base of the lower lashes.

4 **Eye liner:** Take your eye liner brush and wet it. Draw a thin black line at the very base of the upper lashes, starting in the outer corner and gradually making it thinner, so that it's thinnest in the inner corner. Lift the skin of the eye as you're applying it to make sure the line is in the very base of the lashes.

5 **Blush:** Blend a matte pink blush from the cheekbones down the face on a diagonal, stopping on the apples of the cheeks.

6 **Lip color:** Define the lip line with a lip pencil in a color that matches the natural color of the lips. Finish with a berry gloss.

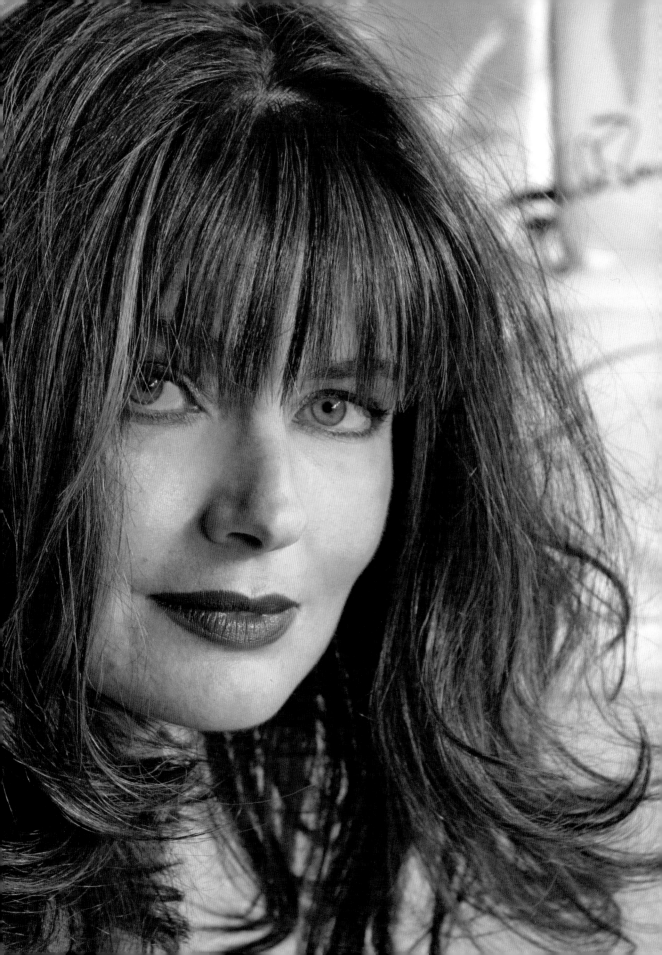

5. glamorous looks

Glamorous color has drama. Even women who are timid about makeup should have some fun and give these looks a try from time to time. Whether you're going out with a group of friends or on a date, these looks are for those occasions when you want to feel—well, glamorous. And if you're feeling starved for attention, a glamorous look will get an immediate reaction from friends and family. Are these looks more complicated or time-consuming? Adding a bright red or ruby red lipstick can immediately give any look more glamour and won't take any extra time at all, but you should set aside more time when you want to perfect your base makeup or apply a stronger eye.

Paulina in a glamorous makeup
that works for day or evening
(see page 136–137 for more on
this look).

accentuating
a face shape

Alva Chinn 50s

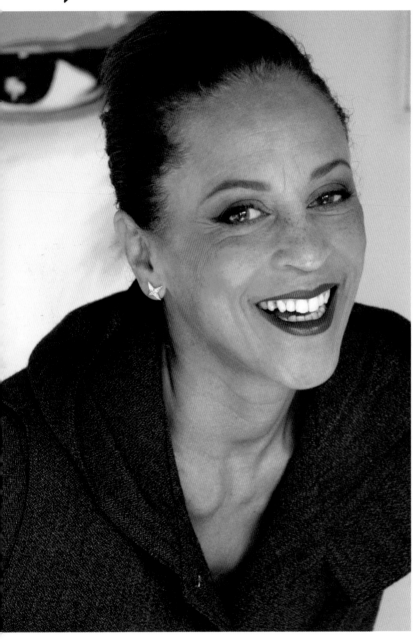

Alva and I met when I first started doing makeup in the late 1970s. As one of the top fashion show models at that time, she was doing all the designer shows during the day while we worked together all night for four nights in a row shooting an advertising campaign. She still models, but acting is now her passion.

For this look, I started with a warm golden yellow liquid base. Because Alva's eyes are round and set deep and close together, I lightened the inner corners with concealer to accentuate them and create the illusion of more space between them. I also used shadows to enlarge and elongate her eyes while accentuating her triangular-shaped face with the diagonal positioning of the blush, which also help to lengthen the eyes visually.

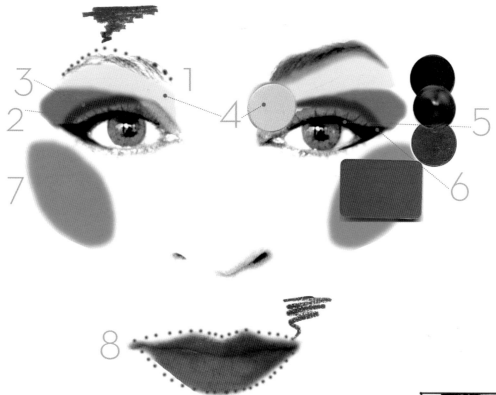

elongated eyes

1 **Eyebrows:** Define with a brunette eyebrow pencil.

2 **Eye shadow/dark tone/accent:** Apply matte olive to the outer two-thirds of the lid, starting at the base of the upper lashes. Blend upward and outward to the crease using the mini-eye shadow brush.

3 **Eye shadow/midtone:** Use the mini-eye shadow brush to heavily apply dark burgundy in the crease, then gently blend it upward and outward toward the end of the brow.

4 **Eye shadow/highlight:** Blend a very light natural matte flesh color on the part of the eyelid near the nose and under the eyebrow.

5 **Eye liner/pencil:** Pencil a brown line at the base of the upper lashes, making sure that it's almost nonexistent in the inner corner but thicker at the outer corner. Dot a little of the same pencil in the outer corner under the eyes, and extend the pencil line upward and outward.

6 **Eye liner/gel/mascara:** Intensify the pencil line at the base of the upper lashes at the outer corners with a dark brown gel liner. Apply black mascara.

7 **Blush:** Add a dash of red powder blush high on the cheekbone. If desired, blend it on the diagonal to accentuate the triangular shape of the face.

8 **Lip color:** Use a brick-colored pencil to outline the lips, slightly building up the upper lip as needed. For long-lasting color, add a soft blue-toned red-brick lip color.

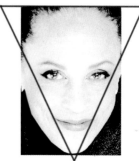

Alva's triangular face shape, which I accentuated to elongate the shape of her round eyes.

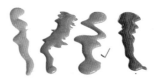

The color of liquid base I chose for Alva's look.

wardrobe inspiration
Diana De Vegh 70s

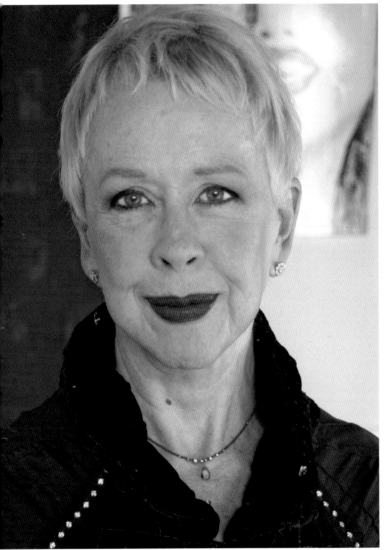

Diana is a psychotherapist in private practice in Greenwich Village. She's also a prototypically doting grandmother who does Pilates twice a week and takes care of her skin by using moisturizers: both a day cream with sunblock, which she's ashamed to say she didn't start wearing until recently, and a night cream. She admits to having had a "nip and tuck," but no shots or peels.

Diana comes to my studio every six months to update her makeup. For our photo shoot, she brought some of her own clothes. She doesn't distinguish between everyday clothes and special-occasion outfits, preferring to dress in her best on a daily basis. "Why not celebrate every day as special and dress accordingly?" she says. I was glad to get a feeling for the colors that Diana wears, to see how she could strengthen her makeup repertoire and enlarge her wardrobe of lip colors. She has a lot of redness in her skin, so I took care of that first, which made it much easier to try different colors.

When Diana changed into a deep burgundy jacket, I felt I needed to make her look stunning, so I added a ruby red lipstick, but then I decided to do a smokier, more neutral eye treatment and also try out a brick color. Diana's lid is smooth, so I can use colors with a slight pearl finish, but definitely not iridescent. She's used to wearing pencil liner in the inner rims of her lower lashes, so we incorporated that into the look I created for her. I didn't add blush because both the eye and the lip are strong, but a light pink powder blush could be brushed lightly on the cheekbones.

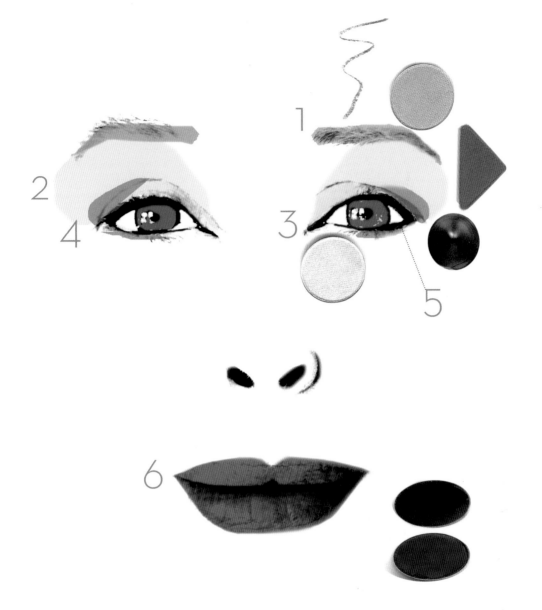

a velvety evening look

1 **Eyebrows:** Define brows with a blond pencil.

2 **Eye shadow/highlight:** Apply a matte beige tint over the brow.

3 **Eye shadow/accent:** Apply a small amount of very pale green to the inner corners of the eyes.

4 **Eye shadow/midtone:** Blend a matte burgundy shadow into the crease and under the eye, blending upward and outward; this will create a slight pink tint in the areas where the burgundy blends with the beige eyeshadow.

5 **Eye liner:** Draw black pencil in the inner rims of the lower lids. Apply black gel eye liner to the base of the upper lashes.

6 **Lip color:** Use brick red for a soft, conservative look, or ruby red for elegance and strength.

BEAUTY CHALLENGE:
evening out redness

Diana's fine skin has a lot of redness, so I applied a liquid base in a very pale color, then a pale cream concealer to cover the redness in her cheeks, and also applied it under her eyes and on her eyelids. A dusting of translucent powder gives the base a longer-lasting finish.

subtle contouring
Anna Bayle 50s

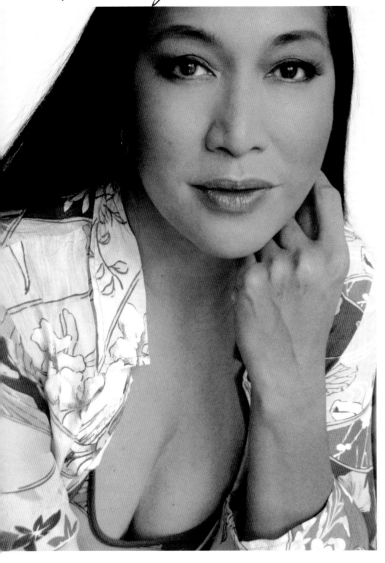

Today Anna Bayle is a writer, but when we first met she was working for all the top designers in Paris, such as Yves Saint Laurent and Thierry Mugler, not just as a model but as their muse and inspiration. Originally from the Philippines, Anna became "the first Asian Supermodel" (according to *The Wall Street Journal*). She began writing about fifteen years ago and now pens articles for fashion magazines and her blog (www.annabayle.com).

Anna has had her makeup done by all the top makeup artists in the world, who've taught her many tricks of the trade. She uses more makeup for going out and likes false eyelashes and a little drama, so I did two different applications on her. For the first look I used only warm colors, which both blended with and brightened her skin tone. Although the eyes are shaded strongly up to the brows, there's an overall softness because all the colors are harmonious, and the false eyelashes accentuate the eyes' upward sweep. To make this look more wearable and modern, I paired it with black lip gloss. This look would also look gorgeous with an orange lip color.

Anna has difficulty finding a base that looks right because of the level of yellow tone in her skin. I found the perfect golden yellow that blended imperceptibly, brightening and slightly evening out her skin tone. This would have been fine for every day, but for a more finished look, I also applied two additional colors of cream base, one three shades darker and one somewhat lighter, to provide more coverage and to contour her face and neck (see page 40 for details).

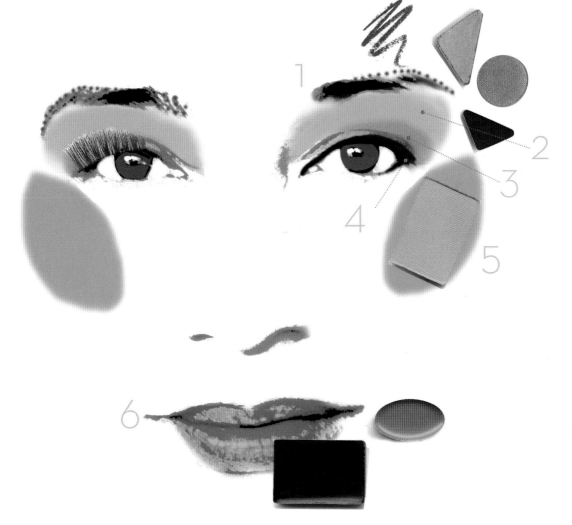

a bright, warm harmony

1 **Eyebrows:** Thicken the eyebrows and fill in any sparse areas with a brunette eyebrow pencil.

2 **Eye shadow/highlight:** Use the large eye shadow brush to blend orange over the brow bone to right under the eyebrow.

3 **Eye shadow/midtone:** Blend a deep green-tinted bronze from the base of the lashes upward and outward in the outer corners of the eyes, going toward the ends of the eyebrows.

4 **Eye liner/mascara/false eyelashes:** Use the eye liner brush and black cake eye liner to line the eyes, making the line thinner in the inner corners. Apply black mascara, then a band of false eyelashes that are longer in the outer corners of the eyes.

5 **Blush:** Blend bright orange powder blush on a diagonal, down over the cheekbones.

6 **Lip color:** For an easy-to-wear look, use just a black lip gloss. For a more finished look, apply a bright orange lip color or a deep brick shade over the gloss.

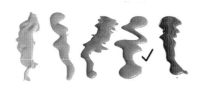

The colors of liquid and cream base I chose for Anna's looks.

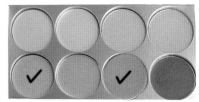

high-contrast eyes

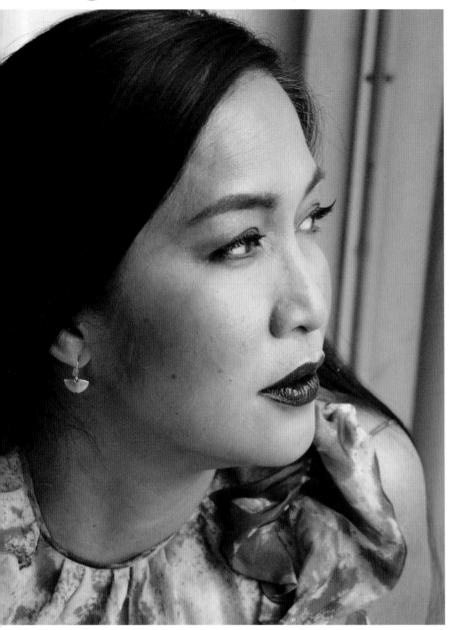

For Anna's second look, I did something a bit more dramatic by choosing a bright, contrasting color for her eyes. I blended in blue-green just past the crease of the eye, which narrowed them and made them more intense; I heightened this effect further by applying no color under the brows. I used the same base colors, contouring, and concealer as I had in the first look (see previous page for details), and false eyelashes again as well.

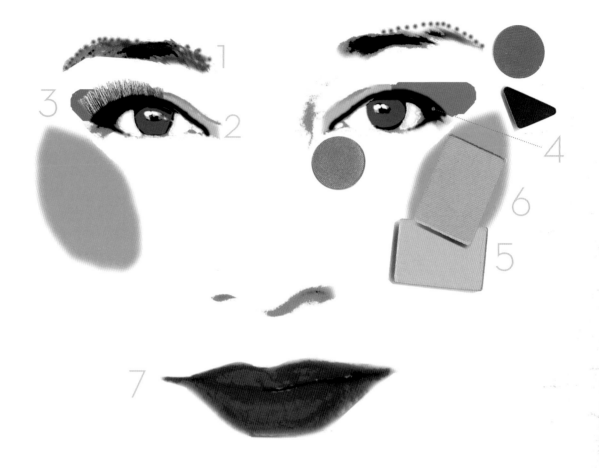

1 **Eyebrows:** Thicken brows and fill in any sparse areas with a brunette pencil.

2 **Eye shadow/accent:** In the inner third of the eyelids, at the base of the lashes, use a mini–eye shadow brush to blend in a green-tinted shiny bronze shadow.

3 **Eye shadow/midtone:** On the outer half of the eyes, press a generous amount of deep jade green into the base of the lashes and blend it straight out, over the crease of the eye (do not blend upward).

4 **Eye liner/false eyelashes:** Line the eyes with a black cake eye liner, extending the line straight out. Use a little at the base of the lower lashes in the outer corner. Apply black false eyelashes to the base of the upper lashes.

5 **Blush:** Blend a light corn shade over the cheekbone and diagonally onto the face.

6 **Blush/accent/powder:** Brighten up and strengthen just the line of the cheekbone with a dot of deeper orange blush. (To blend all the previous products together and to give more matte coverage and color, at this point I used a blusher brush to dust a rich, warm-colored face powder all over Anna's face.)

7 **Lip color:** Apply a deep, rich ruby red.

special occasion
glamour

Barbara Nevins Taylor 50s

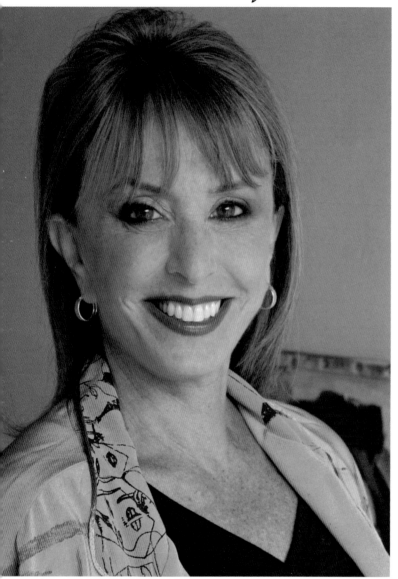

Investigative reporter Barbara Nevins Taylor is passionate about her work. She's had to become skilled at applying her own makeup because a makeup artist isn't always available when she's out working on an assignment.

Although Barbara is fair, with fine skin, I felt that she was a candidate for a warmer base: Her neck and chest are lightly tanned and her personality is warm and outgoing. The medium-warm shade of liquid base was perfect for her because it blends easily for a very natural look and doesn't go on as dark as it looks. I blended the base with a damp sponge, then applied a pale shade of concealer blended over the lid and under the eyes, but only in the inner corners to help create the illusion of space between them.

For a slim face and close-set eyes such as Barbara's, it's important to keep the heaviest part of the eye shading in the outer corner of the eyes and to blend it outward, which appears to lengthen and create space between them. Also, placing the blusher horizontally rounds out the face. Barbara's warm, sparkling personality shines through with a natural look and a soft russet lip color, though stronger lips really accentuate it and also give a glamorous touch—the look she feels the most comfortable with.

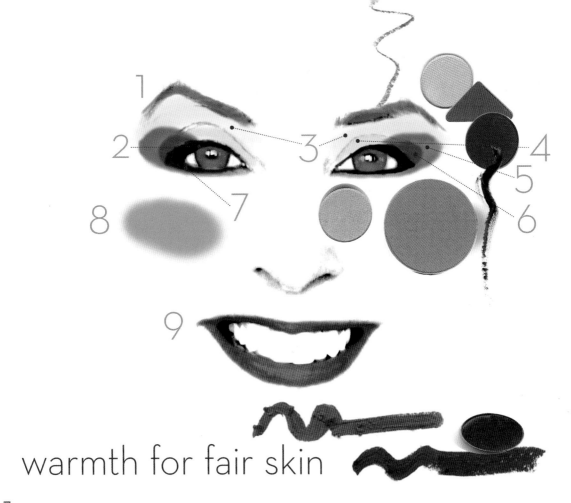

warmth for fair skin

1 **Eyebrows:** Use a blond eyebrow pencil to fill in and define the eyebrows.

2 **Eye liner/translucent powder:** Draw a line at the base of the upper lashes with a black pencil, making it very thin in the inner corner, then thickening it from the center of the eyes outward. Line inside the rim and outside the base of the lower lashes. With a mini-eye shadow brush, extend and blend the line to the outer corners. Press translucent powder onto the line, then powder the rest of the face.

3 **Eye shadow/highlight:** With a large eye shadow brush, blend a pale matte peach over the brow bone.

4 **Eye shadow/accent:** Use the same brush to blend a soft, pale semipearl beige over the inner half of the lid.

5 **Eye shadow/midtone:** With a mini-eye shadow brush, blend a red-brown matte shadow over the penciling under the eyes and in the outer upper crease of the eyes, then blend it into the soft pale peach.

6 **Eye shadow/deep tone:** Using the same brush, press into the base of the lower lashes a dark matte brown. Blend it into the upper outer corner of the eyes at the base of the lashes and outward, into the red-brown.

7 **Eye shadow/liner/mascara:** Press black eye shadow into the base of the lashes to emphasize the penciling. Apply black mascara to both the upper and lower lashes.

8 **Blush:** Blend a matte apricot blush horizontally across the cheeks.

9 **Lip color:** Define with red pencil, then fill in with a bright red or hot pink lip color.

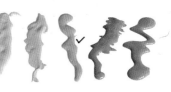

The warm color of liquid base I used on Barbara.

playful charm

Carol Alt / 40s

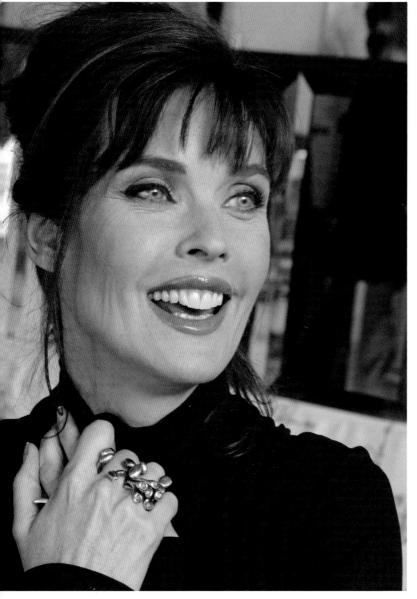

After an enormously successful modeling and acting career, with more than eighteen *Vogue* and *Harper's Bazaar* covers to her credit, Carol has become an amazing entrepreneur with a focus on living a healthy lifestyle. She's an outspoken advocate of a raw food diet and has written two books on the subject, and is also the author of two novels. She also has her own skincare line, Raw Essentials (rawessentials.com), which uses all raw, chemical-free ingredients. Carol's regular makeup routine is simple: If she's going out, she'll wear mascara, lipstick, and maybe a line of black eye liner. She also makes sure to always wear moisturizer.

For this look, I decided to stick with the black eye liner and lengthen the eyes rather like Audrey Hepburn did in the 1960s, with liner in the outer corner of the lower lashes as well as at the base of the upper lashes. For Carol's base, I used a light beige liquid, with concealer only in the inner corners of the eyes and on the lids, followed by a light dusting of translucent powder. If you have fine, dry skin like Carol's, go over the powdering with a damp sponge to take away any excess and give the skin a moister, less made-up look.

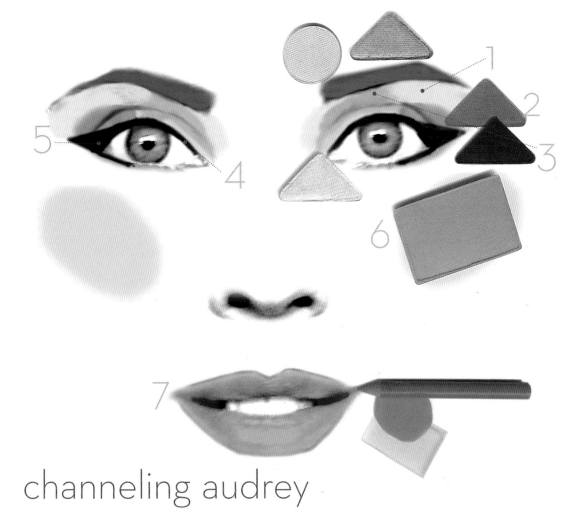

channeling audrey

1 **Eye shadow/highlight:** Create a base for the other shadows by using a large eye shadow brush to blend a light pinky nude matte eye shadow over the entire eyelid.

2 **Eye shadow/midtone:** With a small eye shadow brush, blend a matte gray from the base of the lashes in the outer third of the eye to just past the crease.

3 **Eye shadow/accent:** Use the small eye shadow brush to apply a soft semipearl pink to the crease of the inner corner of the eye, extending it to just under the brow.

4 **Eye shadow/liner:** Apply a very pale soft lilac to the inner corners of the eyes at the base of the lashes using the mini-eye shadow brush or eye liner brush.

5 **Eye liner/mascara:** With a moistened eye liner brush and cake eye liner, draw a short line in the outer corner of each eye at the base of the lower lashes and extend it upward slightly. Draw another line at the base of the upper lashes, thickening it in the outer corner and joining with the extension of the lower line. (Liquid or gel liner could also be used for this step.) Apply lots of black mascara.

6 **Blush:** Blend a matte coral powder blush onto the apples of the cheeks.

7 **Lip color:** Apply a soft pink lip pencil. Over the lip color, apply a nude lip gel (a very light beige with iridescent accents).

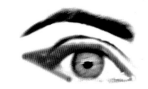

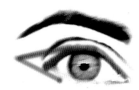

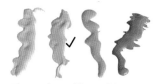

The color of liquid base I chose for Carol.

enjoying it all beautifully
Finn O'Gorman 60s

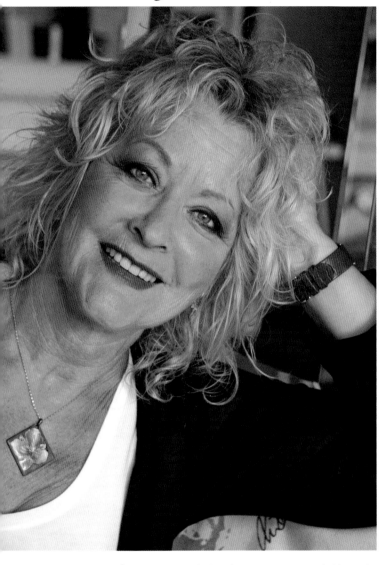

Finn initially came to see me because of a problem with her brows: She had had them tattooed, and now they were becoming faded and gray. I rectified the color loss by applying a matte gold eye shadow with an angled brow brush to warm up their color and make them more natural looking.

Finn loves makeup but thought that as women get older, they have to tone it down. She was happy to learn that this isn't the case. While doing her makeup, we discussed other aspects about her face, such as the white circles around her eyes (a result of wearing glasses for a long time), the pucker lines above her upper lip, and the long hair on her chin. She was very relaxed and had a wonderful attitude ("Use makeup to fix what you can, accept what you can't, and enjoy it!"). I'd heard that lip lines are caused by smoking, so I asked her if she smoked. She said she had stopped smoking more than 30 years ago but believes that the lines are due to her manner of speaking. She explained that she uses her mouth as a French person does, puckering her lips when she makes an *ou* sound. She joked that if she were to adopt a French accent, it would make the lines more acceptable!

I created two looks for Finn that both prove she can still wear strong color. I applied a warm base over her entire face to maintain her tan and tone down any redness and then applied a slightly darker one around the eyes to minimize the lightness there. To make sure that her lip color didn't bleed, I used matte lipsticks and soft pencil liners, then powdered the outline to set it.

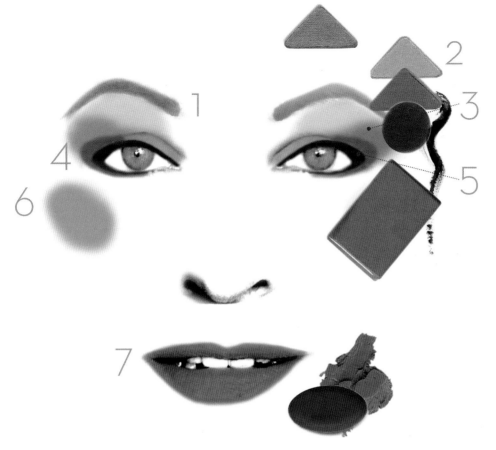

finished elegance and strength

1 **Eyebrows:** Using an angled brow brush, blend a matte gold eye powder over the brows.

2 **Eye shadow/highlight:** With a large eye shadow brush, blend in a soft, semipearl peach shade over the entire eyelid.

3 **Eye shadow/midtone:** With your small eye shadow brush, blend in a red-brown matte eye shadow over the peach shadow at the base of the lashes. Blend it over the crease from the center of the eyes outward, toward the ends of the brows.

4 **Eye liner:** Line the base of the upper lashes with a black eye liner pencil. Apply a small amount to the outer corners of the eyes at the base of the lower lashes.

5 **Eye shadow/deep tone/mascara:** With your mini–eye shadow brush, press a matte dark brown eye shadow powder onto the black penciling at the base of both the upper and lower lashes; then blend it into the red-brown area, just past the crease of the eye in the outer corner. Apply black mascara to both the upper and lower lashes.

6 **Powder/Blush:** Set the makeup at this point by dabbing translucent powder all over the face, paying special attention to the nose, forehead, and chin. Blend a matte russet shade of blush diagonally on the cheekbone, tapering off at the apples of the cheeks.

7 **Lip color:** Apply a muted lip color to the lips, then define them by outlining them with deeper red lip shade; blend the two colors together. If needed, finish by powdering the edges of the lips.

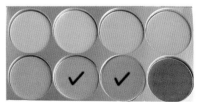

The colors of cream base I chose for Finn's looks.

flirtatious lilac and hot pink

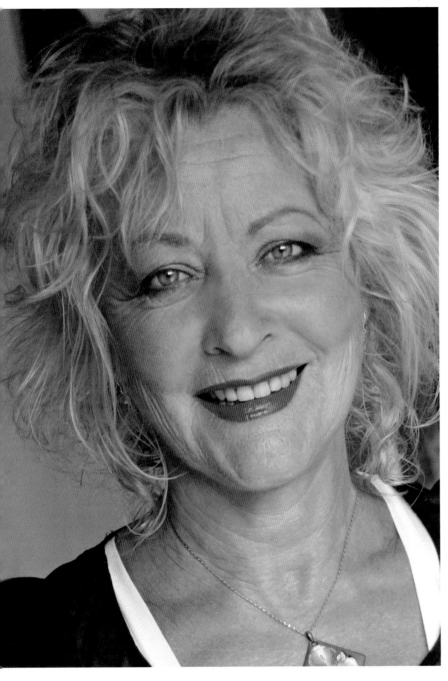

This look could easily become too "made-up," but to make the contrasting violet hues easier to wear, I kept the blush in the same warm tonality and simply strengthened the eyes and lips so they would stand out in contrast. I used the same base, concealer, and brows as for Finn's previous look.

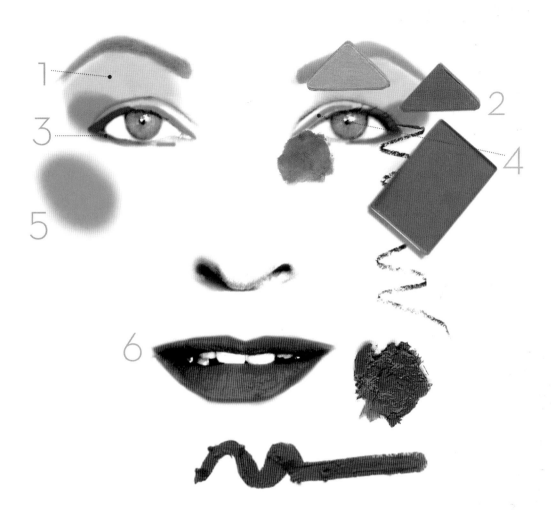

1 **Eye shadow/highlight:** With a large eye shadow brush, blend a soft, semipearl peach shade over the entire eyelid.

2 **Eye shadow/midtone:** With a small eye shadow brush, blend red-brown matte eye shadow into the outer corners of the eyes, away from and over the creases.

3 **Eye liner:** Line the base of the upper lashes with a thin line of brown pencil, keeping the liner very thin in the inner corners of the eyes. Apply a small amount to the outer corners of the eyes at the base of the lower lashes.

4 **Eye shadow/accent/mascara:** With a mini-eye shadow brush, press iridescent violet powder eye shadow into the inner corners of the eyes at the base of both upper and lower lashes; blend in lightly. Apply black mascara to both the upper and lower lashes.

5 **Powder/blush:** Set the makeup with a dusting of translucent powder all over the face, paying special attention to the nose, forehead, and chin. Blend a matte russet blush diagonally on the cheekbone, tapering off at the apples of the cheeks.

6 **Lip color:** Apply hot pink lip color with a lip brush; then define by outlining with pink lip pencil. Powder the edges of the lips with translucent powder.

a hard rocker's softer side

Joan Jett 50s

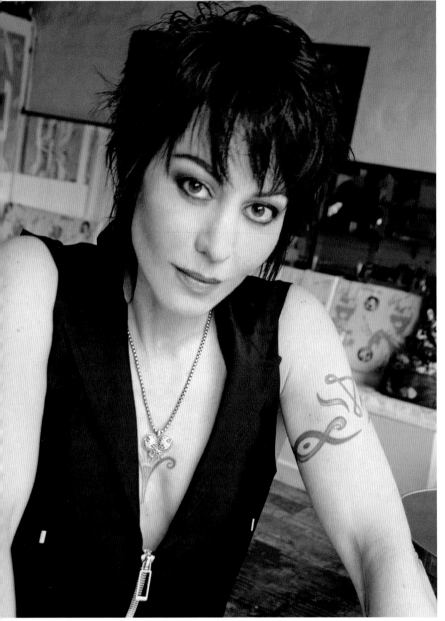

Rock star Joan Jett enjoys getting her makeup done and finds it relaxing. Her everyday makeup ranges from basic to more extreme, and she regularly wears black eye liner. On stage she wears blended dark colors and sometimes lighter ones. She's learned a great deal about makeup over the years and loved the look she wore while doing *The Rocky Horror Picture Show* on Broadway. There was "no holding back," and she felt she went outside of herself with her dramatic makeup of neon greens, blue glitter, and other dazzling colors and effects. I was flattered when she said that her most memorable makeup experience was when I painted her freestyle for her *FlashBack* album cover.

No one has seen Joan in very soft makeup, so I wanted show how her great features "pop" with just a subtle application of color and a slight evening out of her skin (see page 51 for this look). I used the same base for both looks, but for this one I added drama with darker eye liner and contrasting brown and white eye shadow.

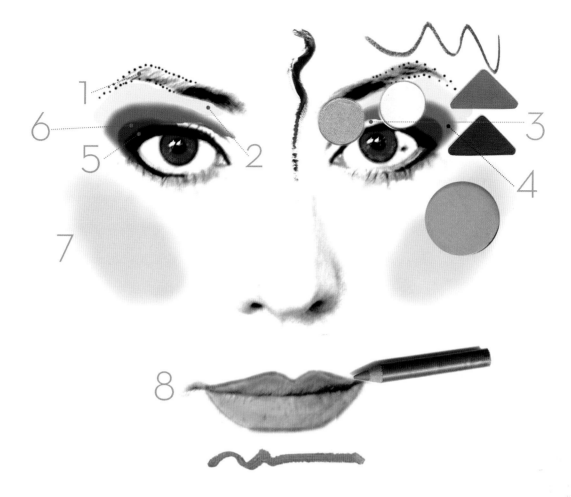

wearable glam rock

1 **Eyebrows**: Strengthen the apex and ends of the brows with a dark brown pencil.

2 **Eye shadow/highlight:** Dust a matte white shadow over the eyelids from the lashes to the brows.

3 **Eye shadow/accent:** Use an eye liner brush to apply silver shadow to the eyelids.

4 **Eye shadow/midtone:** Apply matte warm brown shadow to the creases of the eyes, going over onto the brow bones.

5 **Eye liner:** Line the base of the upper lashes with black pencil, making sure the line is thinner in the inner corners and thicker in the outer corners. Apply the pencil very gently under the inner corners of the lower lashes, then thicken it toward the outer corners. Blend the upper and lower lines together.

6 **Eye shadow/deep tone/mascara:** Press matte black eye shadow onto the pencil under and above the eyes. Blend the black shadow into the outer crease, applying it heavily and partially covering the brown to create an uplifting oval shape in the outer areas of the eyes. Apply black mascara.

7 **Blush:** Blend dusty pink blush from the cheekbone down the face on a diagonal.

8 **Lip color:** Apply a soft pink lipstick, then define the lips with a muted pink lip pencil.

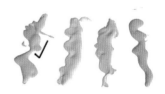

The color of liquid base I used on Joan.

embracing glamour
Debbie Dickinson 50s

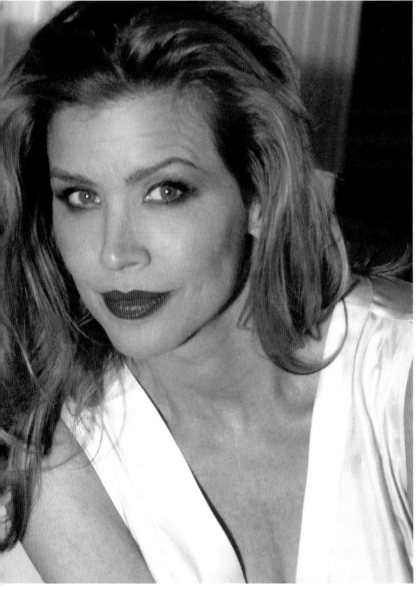

Debbie Dickinson was the first Victoria's Secret model and continues her modeling career, along with her work as an actress and entrepreneur (she has her own public relations firm). As a wearer of many hats in her professional life, she highly recommends versatility and playing with makeup. Her mottos are, "Your image gives you an important edge in business," and "Beauty is power." She sometimes has her makeup professionally applied for her business meetings, depending on her audience. As she puts it, "Makeup is my best friend."

Though in the 1970s Debbie regularly wore glitz makeup and rainbow colors, her current everyday makeup routine is much simpler. She uses a moisturizing compact foundation and a little cream blush: pinks in the winter, corals in the summer. She wears powder, but not on the cheeks.

Debbie inspired me to do a glamorous makeup look, enlarging and lengthening her round eyes (see page 58 for details) and accentuating her fabulous lips with a beautiful red. For her base makeup, I applied a light shade of cream base with a damp sponge over her entire face, blending concealer in one shade lighter around her eyes, especially in the inner corners. I finished with a light dusting of translucent powder, applying it a bit more heavily around the nose and chin.

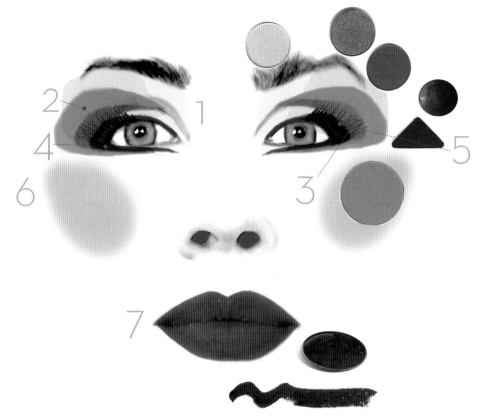

enlarging and lifting round eyes

1 **Eye shadow/highlight:** With a small eye shadow brush, apply a matte vanilla eye shadow to the inner corners of the eyes.

2 **Eye shadow/midtone:** With a large eye shadow brush, apply a wash of a deep, slightly iridescent plum hue from the base of the lashes to the outer ends of the brows. Using the small eye shadow brush, apply the same shadow more heavily, starting under the eye, then extending it and sweeping it around, into and past the crease.

3 **Eye shadow/deep tone:** With a mini–eye shadow brush, blend a deep matte burgundy shadow under the eye at the very base of the lower lashes, extending the eye shape with the shadow and going very heavily into the crease. This application will visually lower the inner corners and lift the outer corners of the eyes.

4 **Eye shadow/accent:** With the side of a mini–eye shadow brush, blend black eye shadow into the base of the lower lashes. As with the burgundy shadow, depart from the lash base in the inner corner and extend the color to the outer corner, blending the black shadow at the outer top corner of the eye, from the lashes to the crease.

5 **Eye liner/false eyelashes:** Apply black or deep blue green liner to the base of the upper lashes. To further lengthen the eyes and give them a natural upsweep, apply three or four clusters of medium eyelashes to the very base of the upper lashes in the outer corners.

6 **Blush:** Dust a soft, warm peach matte powder blusher on the cheekbones, blending it downward onto the apples of the cheeks.

7 **Lip color:** Apply a stunning red with a slight shine.

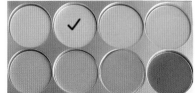

The color of cream base I chose for Debbie.

true beauty, inside and out

Paulina Porizkova 40s

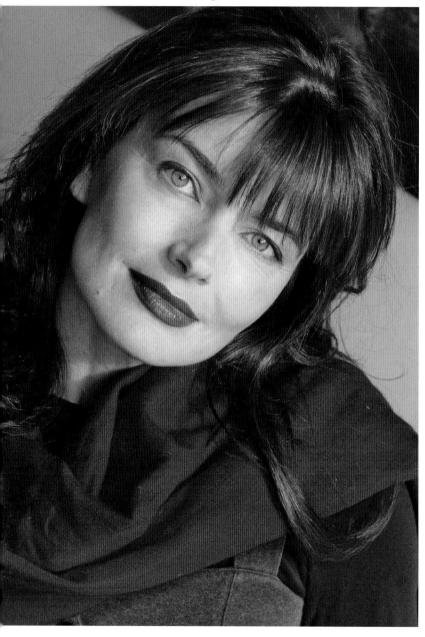

I remember vividly the very first job I did with Paulina at the beginning of the 1980s, when she first started modeling in Paris, just before I moved to New York. She's always inspired me: She's both beautiful and photogenic, with the most amazing skin and bone structure. Her skin hasn't changed—it's still as luminous as ever—so I just applied a thin layer of light beige liquid base with a damp sponge, then blended a little light cream concealer to her lids and under her eyes.

If you have great skin and a fabulous lip shape, red lipstick is a fast way to glamorize your face. If you feel the red to be overpowering after you've applied it, you can strengthen the eyes slightly by adding a soft mushroom-colored shadow to the lids, starting at the crease and blending it gently outward and then adding lots of mascara.

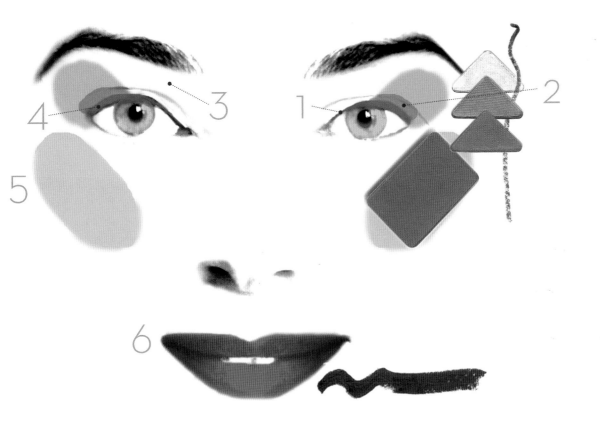

drop-dead gorgeous

1 **Eye liner:** Apply a small amount of gray pencil to the very base of the upper outer lashes.

2 **Eye shadow/accent:** With a mini–eye shadow brush, press a soft matte gray shadow onto the penciling and blend it up onto the lid just enough to accentuate the shape of the eyes.

3 **Eye shadow/highlight:** With a large eye shadow brush, dust a soft iridescent gold-tinted white shadow over the entire eyelid.

4 **Eye shadow/midtone/mascara:** With the small eye shadow brush, blend a soft semipearl beige from the outer half of the eye upward and outward. Apply mascara generously.

5 **Blush:** Apply a matte red blush to the apples of the cheeks.

6 **Lip color:** With great skin and a fabulous lip shape, a stunning red is a fast way to glamorize your face. To look like a fashion model, leave it heavy and shiny; for less impact, tone it down by blotting it with a tissue.

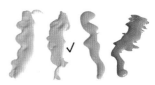

The color of liquid base I used for Paulina's looks.

gala event

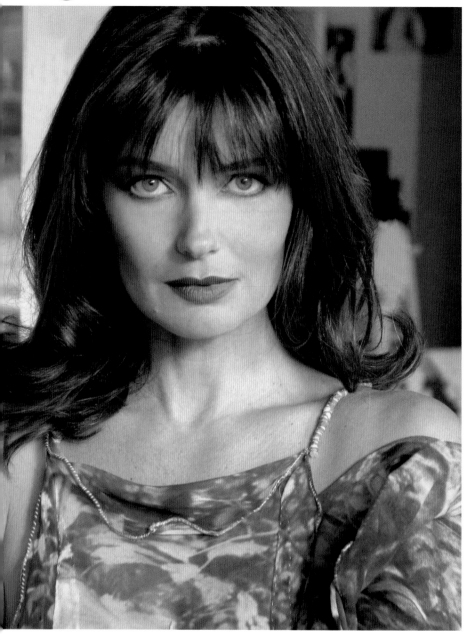

For this look, I kept Paulina's skin tone the same, strengthened the color of her eyes and cheeks, and softened her lips by using a slightly less vibrant red. I lined her eyes heavily with a hunter green pencil, then blended the pencil into the crease of the eye, applying a jade green eye shadow over it. The jade green was blended into the soft semipearl beige I had applied under the eyebrow. To soften the undereye pencil, apply a light beige matte shadow over it.

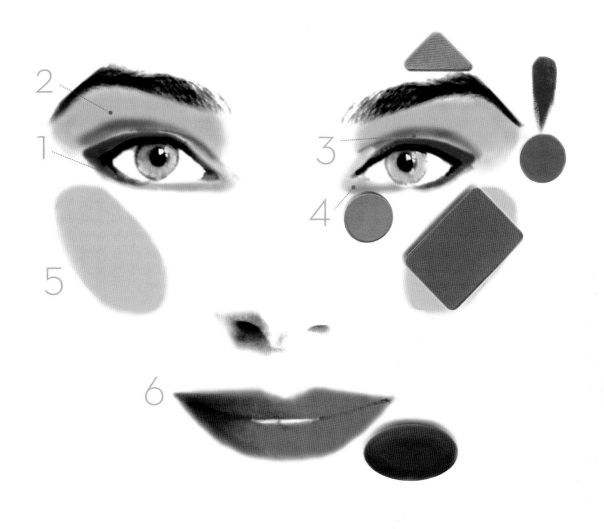

1 **Eye liner:** Line the eyes heavily with a dark green pencil, then blend the line into the creases.

2 **Eye shadow/highlight:** Blend a soft semipearl beige under the eyebrow and over the brow bone using a large eye shadow brush.

3 **Eye shadow/deep tone:** Blend jade green eye shadow over the penciling and into the soft, shimmery beige applied under the eyebrow.

4 **Eye shadow/shading/mascara:** To soften the undereye pencil line, apply a light beige matte shadow over it. Finish the eyes with black mascara.

5 **Blush:** Blend a matte pink over the cheekbones on a diagonal.

6 **Lip color:** Use a soft matte red very lightly, or blot down a bright red and rub a little pink into it.

active glamour
Barbara Novogratz 70s

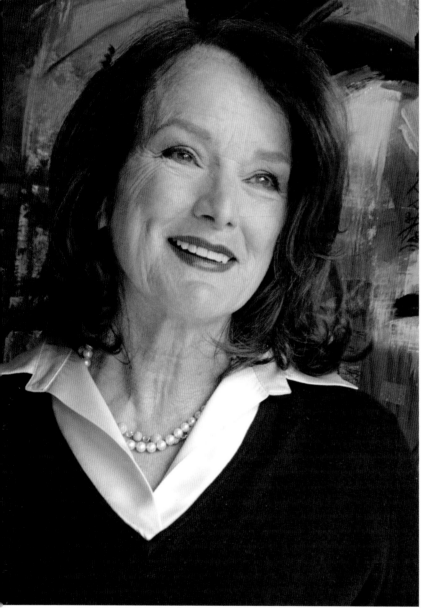

Barbara is an antiques dealer and leads a very busy life. She's constantly traveling for her business as well as visiting her many children and grandchildren. She never goes out without her makeup, and she always looks great when I see her.

When Barbara arrived for our session, she was wearing a very fine base that suited her perfectly, so all I did was give a little more coverage with a light shade of cream base down the sides of the nose and on the chin, where there was slight redness. I also very lightly applied a light shade of concealer to the inner corners of her eyes and on her eyelids. I was very careful not to overdo the blush, as Barbara has strong, beautiful cheekbones, so I used a matte powder blush very sparingly; anything shiny would have accentuated them too much.

Barbara's main complaint is that her eye makeup seems to run under her eyes, which I showed her how to avoid (see Beauty Challenge, opposite). Barbara's lips are quite asymmetrical and not well defined, so it's important for her to follow the steps on page 77 to correct the asymmetry.

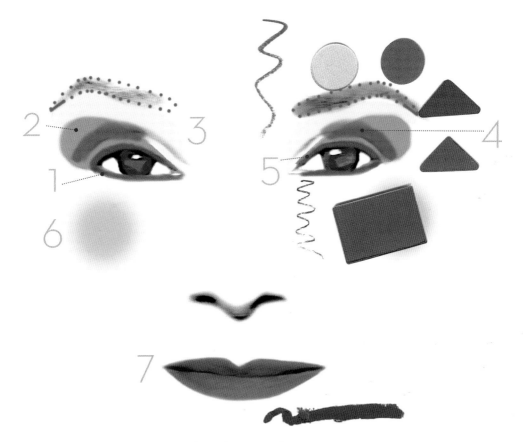

pretty and polished

1 **Eyebrows/pencil liner:** Define the brows with brown pencil, then apply it at the base of the lower lashes and blend it lightly with the mini–eye shadow brush.

2 **Eye shadow/midtone:** With the large eye shadow brush, blend matte olive eye shadow from the base of the upper lashes past the crease of the eye. Go over the crease with more of the olive shadow to strengthen it, using the mini-eye shadow brush. Blend a little of the same shadow with the mini-eye shadow brush over the brown penciling under the eye, at the base of the lower lashes.

3 **Eye shadow/highlight:** Use a large eye shadow brush to blend matte vanilla eye shadow from the inner corners of the eyes onto the brow bones.

4 **Eye shadow/accent:** With a small eye shadow brush, press matte red-brown eye shadow into the crease at the center of the eye, moving the brush back and forth over the olive shadow in this area to intensify the color. At this point you can set the undereye makeup with translucent powder (see Beauty Challenge, at right).

5 **Eye liner:** Line the base of the upper lashes with a soft red-brown eye liner using an eye liner brush.

6 **Blush:** Brush a touch of russet blush onto the cheekbones.

7 **Lip color:** Define the lips with a lip brush and burgundy lip color. Add a touch of gloss to the center of the lips.

BEAUTY CHALLENGE:
runny eye makeup

To keep Barbara's eye makeup from running, I showed her how to press a little translucent powder onto the shading under the eyes with the point of a clean, wide, firm eye shadow brush, then to dust the powder lightly over her undereye concealer.

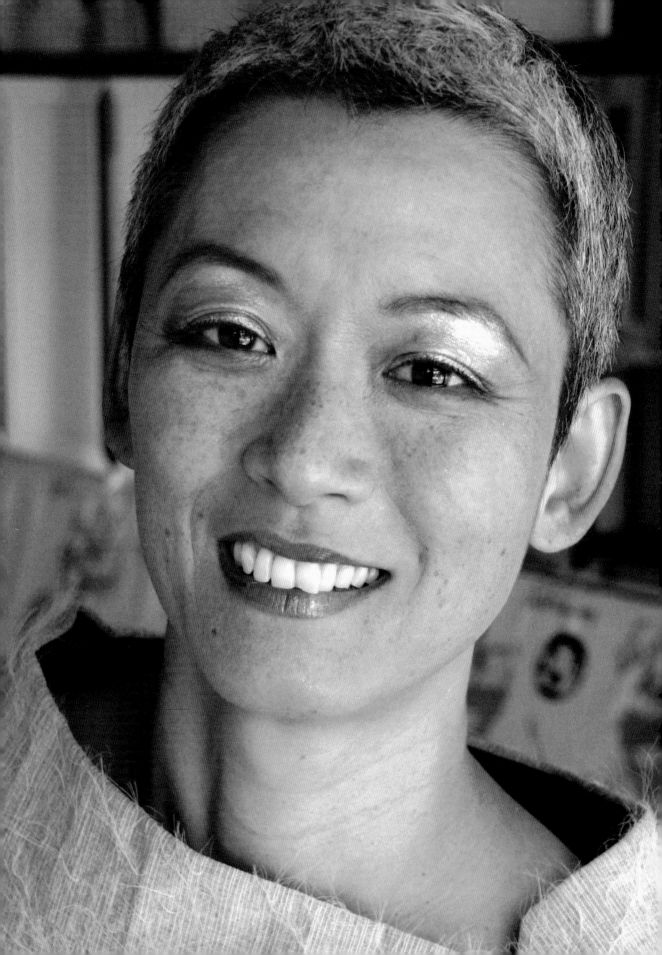

6. creative looks

Creative looks are daring and expressive, but not overpowering. The key
is to be just bold enough to buy a few colors you love and take the time to
experiment. As the looks in this chapter show, with adventurous undertakings
come big payoffs: Creative color can transform a face into a piece of art and
accentuate your personality.

Artist Mimi Oka enjoys
experimenting with makeup
(see page 150–151 for details
on this look).

elegant personal touches
Cécile Defforey 60s

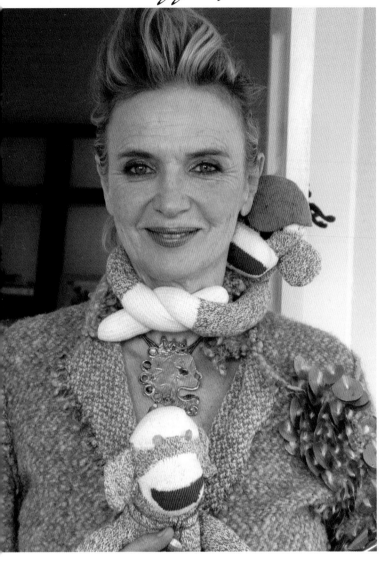

This book wouldn't be complete without someone from the beauty capital of the world: Paris. Cécile is an artist and the epitome of the enigmatic, alluring Frenchwoman. Everything she does seems to enhance her beauty. I began our session with a pared-down, natural look (see page 22). Cécile's reaction? She felt naked! Even for every day, Cécile uses a brighter lip color and adds allure to her eyes with blue pencil applied to the inner rims of her lower lashes; she then blends it slightly outward like Cleopatra, enhancing her almond-shaped eyes. For this colorful look, I merely expanded on that approach with an extra boost of color. Cécile also makes beautiful pieces of jewelry, and here she is wearing one of her favorite pieces, which just happens to replicate her favorite makeup colors.

For Cécile's base makeup, I started with a very lightweight liquid base with a slight yellow undertone and added a light concealer to darker areas such as larger freckles. Her brows are fading a little, so I filled in the sparse areas with a blond pencil. I applied a strongly pearlized deep-aqua shadow to the very base of her lashes, then a deeper blue-green to the inner rims and the bases of the lower lashes. I used a little matte gray in the outer corners to strengthen them and a touch of white shimmer in the inner corner of her eyes. Then I used lots of black mascara. Cécile has very thick lashes, which she cuts from time to time. I finished the look with a coral blush and a soft coral lip color.

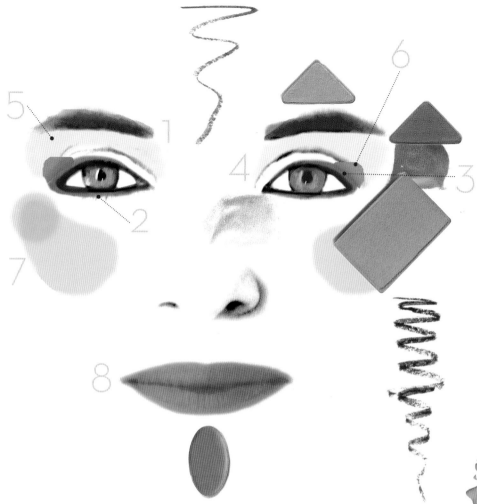

The color of liquid base I used on Cécile.

dramatic shimmer

1 **Eyebrows:** Strengthen brows as needed with a blond eyebrow pencil.

2 **Eye liner pencil:** Apply a deep blue-green pencil inside the rims and to base of the lower lashes. Blend the liner beneath the eyes with a mini-eye shadow brush.

3 **Eye liner/shadow:** Use the mini-eye shadow brush to press an iridescent aqua shade into the base of the upper lashes.

4 **Eye shadow/highlight:** Using the eye liner brush, apply white pearl shadow to the inner corners of the eyes at the base of the lashes.

5 **Eye shadow/accent:** Brush a soft peach eye shadow lightly over the brow bones. Finish the eyes by generously applying black mascara.

6 **Eye shadow/accent:** Apply a matte gray shadow to the outer corners of the eyes and blend it just past the crease.

7 **Blush:** Brush a coral blusher onto the cheeks.

8 **Lip color:** Apply a soft coral lip color with a lip brush.

BEAUTY CHALLENGE:
making up eyes with fine lines

I usually advise older women to avoid eye shadows with shine because they accentuate lines on the lids and around the eyes. However, if placed right next to the lashes, they can be very flattering, especially on an eye shape like Cécile's, as she has very little room between the base of her lashes and her brows. So she's an ideal candidate for color and shine at the base of her lashes and liner applied inside and under the eyes.

balancing eyes, lips, and cheeks

Grisel Baltazar 40s

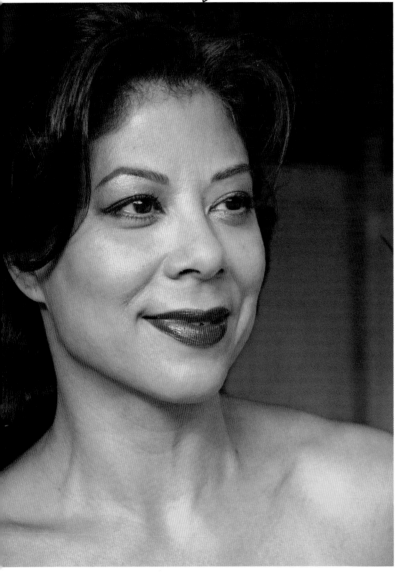

Grisel, who's a teacher, has always loved makeup. When she was younger she simply wore what she liked, but she came to me because she felt she no longer knew how to wear it.

Grisel told me that base was her most difficult makeup challenge. She wanted the smooth finish of a cream base but thought it looked too heavy. We decided to use a medium shade of gel base (she is wearing this on page 39), which evened out Grisel's skin slightly, making it matte and clean looking. But the gel base was too fine to provide the coverage she needed on the darker areas of her face, so I blended two warm shades of cream base around her mouth and under her eyes and added concealer to the inner corners of her eyes, then finished with a light dusting of translucent powder.

As a departure from the more discreet makeup I created for her to wear while she's teaching, which features a matte violet eye (see pages 68-69), I designed a look that combined strong lips with iridescent violet shadows on her eyes, which worked beautifully on her smooth lids; I balanced the two by using no blush. Iridescent shadows are very pretty when judiciously applied, but they must be dusted over matte shadows of the same color with a large eye shadow brush in order to give the eye depth.

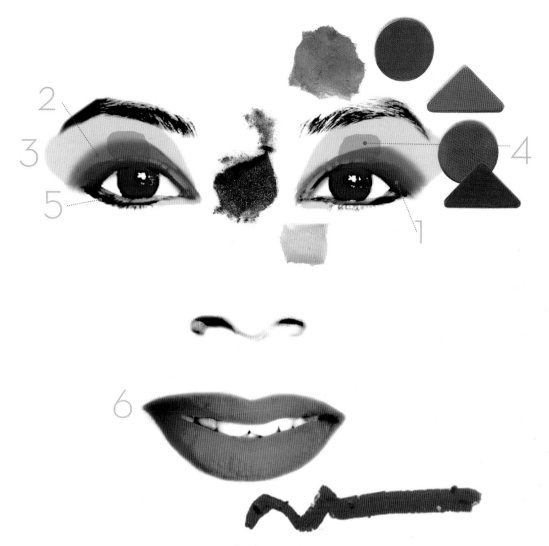

strong eyes and lips

1 **Eye shadow/deep tone:** Apply a deep matte purple shadow to the base of the lashes in the outer part of the eye, blending it outward and upward.

2 **Eye shadow/midtone:** Blend a matte violet shadow in the crease, also in the outer part of the eye.

3 **Eye shadow/highlight:** Use a large eye shadow brush to dust iridescent lilac shadow over the entire eyelid.

4 **Eye shadow/accent:** Press a sparkly violet shadow onto the center of the eyelid.

5 **Eye liner:** Apply a thin line of a deep violet eye liner to the base of the upper lashes, making the line thinner in the inner corners. Add a little of the liner to the base of the lower lashes.

6 **Lip color:** Apply a vibrant blue-red with a lip brush. Add an accent of white iridescent eye shadow to the bow of the lips.

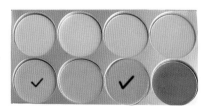

The colors of cream base I used on Grisel.

bringing cheeks into play

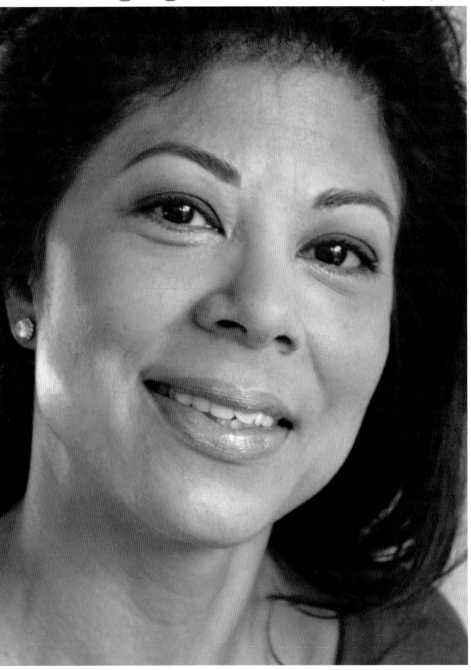

For this look, I wanted to shift the emphasis from the lips not just by using a subtle lip color but by softening the eyes with matte shadows and adding a sweep of coral blush. I created a smooth foundation by applying the two cream bases over Grisel's face and eyelids, then a slightly lighter shade of concealer around her eyes.

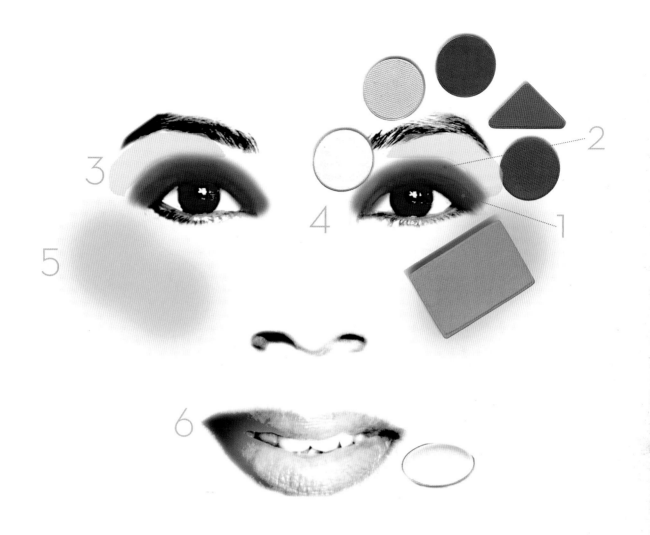

1 **Eye shadow/deep tone:** Use the mini-eye shadow brush to press deep purple matte shadow into the very base of the upper lashes and blend it onto the lid and upward past the crease of the eye.

2 **Eye shadow/midtone/translucent powder:** Press a brighter matte violet into the crease of the eye. Powder the face and eyes (over the shadows) with translucent powder.

3 **Eye shadow/highlight:** Brush a matte light pink over the brow bone with a large eye shadow brush.

4 **Eye shadow/accent (optional):** Apply matte white to the inner corners of the eyes and iridescent white to the base of the lower lashes.

5 **Blush:** Apply a coral powder blush (which I applied to Grisel's cheek's diagonally).

6 **Lip color:** Apply lip gloss in subtle white pearl.

enhancing green eyes

Lilo Zinglersen 50s

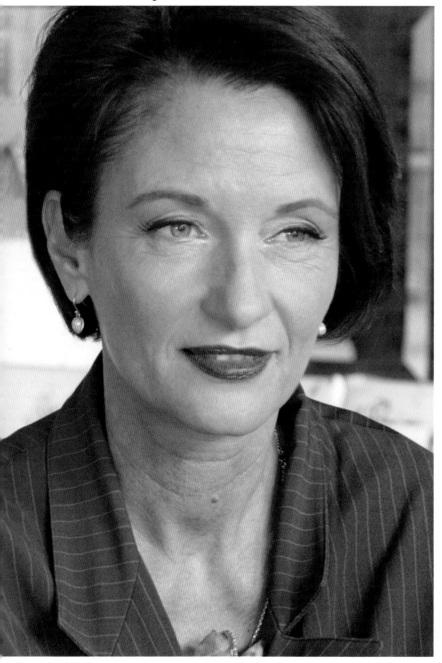

Lilo is a natural beauty who modeled during the late 1970s and '80s in both Europe and the United States. She was high energy and lots of fun to work with. These days, Lilo channels that energy into horse breeding and training, for which she wears little makeup. Most of her makeup is geared toward special occasions, when she goes for a stronger, more compelling look. For her creative color makeup, we went with a strong eye to play up her fabulous green eyes. For the base, I used a warm beige cream base to cover red areas, applying transparent powder lightly, using a cotton powder puff over the entire face and a small powder brush around the nose and chin.

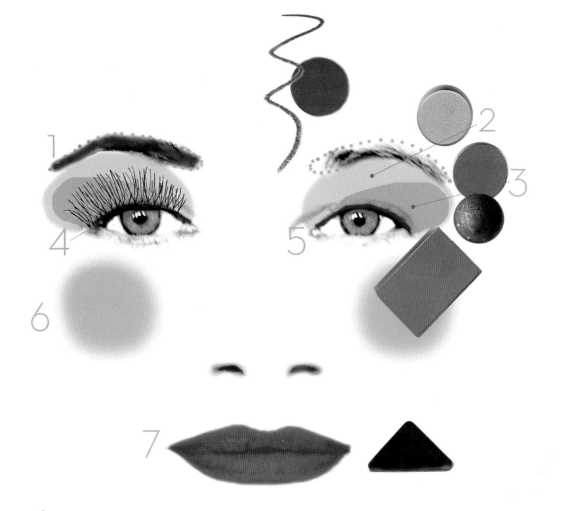

going green

1 **Eyebrows:** Fill in and even out brows with a blond pencil using small strokes, then brush lightly with the spiral brow brush. Blend in dark brown powder shadow with an angled brow brush. Finish with the spiral brush.

2 **Eye shadow/highlight:** Using a large eye shadow brush, blend a lime eye shadow powder over the entire eyelid, from the base of the lashes to the brow.

3 **Eye shadow/midtone:** Blend jade green from the base of the lashes outward toward the ends of the brows.

4 **Eye liner:** Use an eye liner brush to cover the base of the upper lashes with a very thin line of green gel eye liner.

5 **Eye shadow/accent/mascara/lashes:** Add a touch of very pale green iridescent eye shadow to the inner corners of the eyes at the very base of both the upper and lower lashes. Apply lots of black mascara, then add a band of widely spaced false eyelashes to the base of the upper lashes.

6 **Blush:** Blend a warm russet shade of powder blush onto the apples of the cheeks, no closer in than the center of the eye.

7 **Lip color:** Apply a brick red lip color.

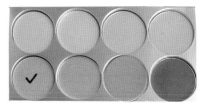

The color of cream base I chose for Lilo.

BEAUTY CHALLENGE:
sparse lashes

For Lilo I opted for a band of black false eyelashes that were spaced out to give the effect of individually placed lashes. This type of false eyelashes is easier to apply than individual ones and can be taken off and worn a few times.

expanding
artistic expression
Mimi Oka 50s

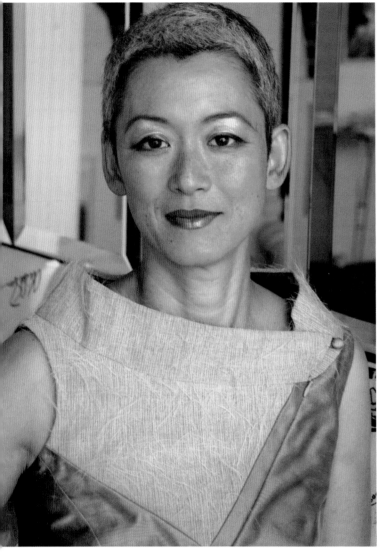

Mimi is an artist who until a few years ago didn't wear makeup. As she matured and her career expanded, she had more art events and openings to attend. She eventually realized that makeup wasn't just about enhancing looks but also a legitimate tool for artistic expression and for feeling good about oneself.

To help Mimi become comfortable with the idea of applying makeup (I didn't want her to feel that it was in any way masklike), and because she had fairly even skin tone, initially I avoided base and concealer and just concentrated on playing with color. I did simple things, such as applying touches of bright-colored cream shadows or liner and a black lip gloss to deepen her lip color. I kept it all very playful and easy to change.

Although I had at first avoided applying base and concealer, there were times when I felt her skin needed brightening up. So I taught her how to blend two colors of a very lightweight liquid base in the same undertone as her skin but slightly lighter in color with a damp sponge until it was imperceptible, then to tap a little concealer onto the lids and under the eyes to lighten those areas as well.

As I continued to work on her, I was amazed at how good she looked in a variety of different makeup styles—bright lips, dark eyes, false eyelashes, even adjusting the shape and color of her brows. Over the course of a couple of private lessons, I've shown Mimi how to create many different looks so that now she isn't afraid to try anything.

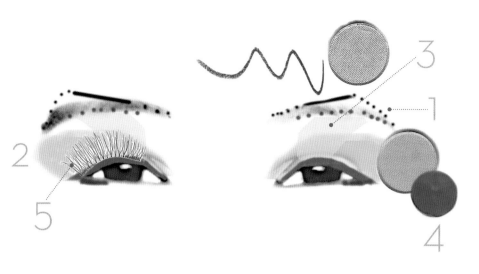

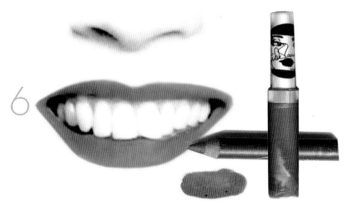

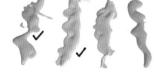

The false eyelashes I applied to Mimi. The base of these brown lashes is almost colorless, which makes them soft and easy to wear.

The colors of liquid base I used on Mimi.

stylishly creative

1 **Eyebrows:** Define the brows as needed with a blond eyebrow pencil.

2 **Eye shadow/midtone:** Use a small eye shadow brush to apply lime green matte shadow from the base of the lashes toward the outer part of the eyebrows.

3 **Eye shadow/highlight:** With a large eye shadow brush, dust bright silver shadow onto the center of the eyelid, from the crease to the brows.

4 **Eye liner:** Line the eyes with a bright blue liner.

5 **False eyelashes:** Use very lightweight brown lashes.

6 **Lip color:** Define the lips with a muted pink and finish with a deep lilac gloss.

BEAUTY CHALLENGE:
prominent eye fold

Because Mimi's eye fold is almost on top of her lashes, it's important that she extend any color she applies both above and below it. I had her apply touches of color to her lid with her eyes open, extending it past the eye fold, and then close her eye and blend the color downward to the lashes.

easy creative

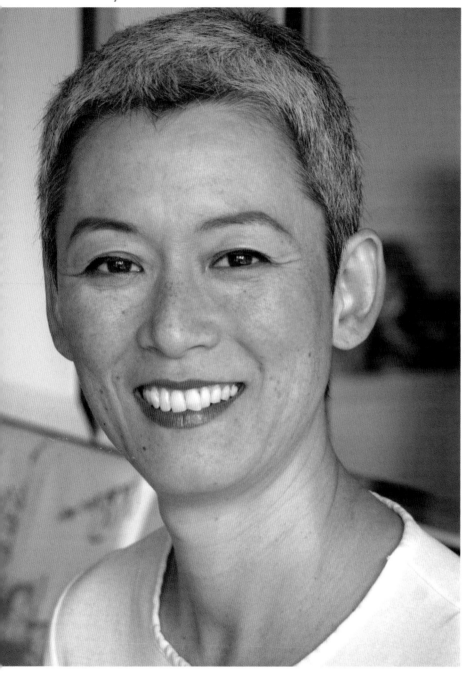

What could be simpler than one eye shadow with some eye liner? Try any mixture of bright or unusual shadow colors with liner: If red is too daring for you, try violet. Note that here Mimi is only wearing concealer and a little powder, no base.

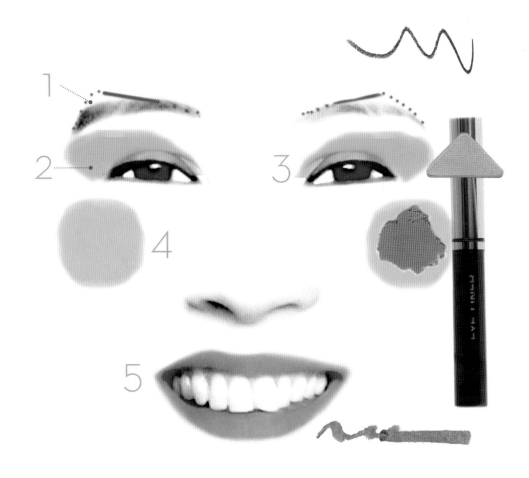

1 **Eyebrows:** Define the brows as needed with a blond eyebrow pencil.

2 **Eye shadow:** Using the small eye shadow brush, apply a yellow, sand-colored matte eye shadow from the base of the lashes, blending so that there's no color just under the eyebrows.

3 **Eye liner:** Highlight the eyes with a very thin line of red. If you prefer a lighter look, keep the liner very thin for the first two-thirds of the eye and thicken it at the end.

4 **Blush:** Dot the cheeks with a pink cream blush and blend well.

5 **Lip color:** Apply a creamy peach lip gloss.

bright eyes and lips

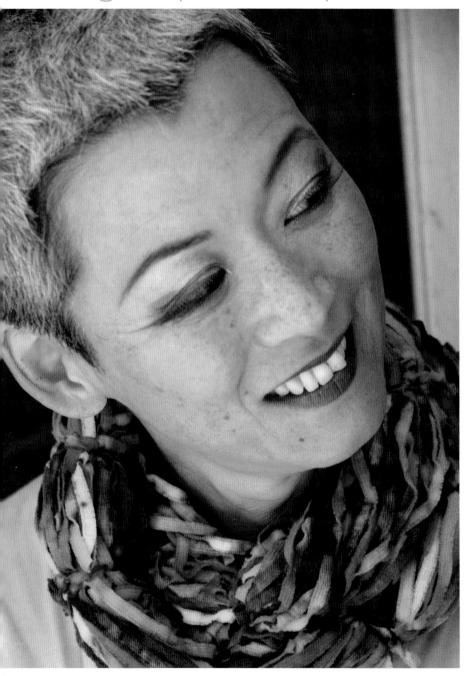

This combination of colors is very easy to wear as long as you don't wear blush and keep the warm color on the eyes the same as that on the lips. The base and concealer are the same as for the first look, but this time I finished with a dusting of translucent powder over the entire face before applying the eyes, cheeks, and lips.

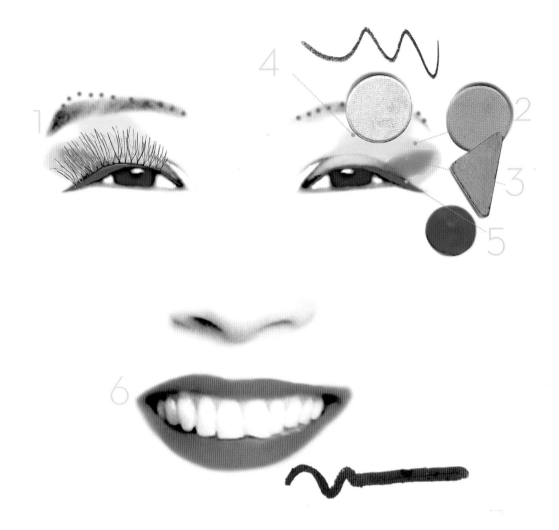

1 **Eyebrows:** Define and lengthen the brows as needed with a thinly drawn blond eyebrow pencil line.

2 **Eye shadow/midtone:** Use a small eye shadow brush to dot a lime-green eye shadow, starting from the outer corner of the eyelids and blending it upward and outward toward the outer brows.

3 **Eye shadow/accent:** Press bright orange shadow into a smaller area within the lime-green shadow. If you find the color isn't vivid enough, dab some yellow or orange cream shadow or a tiny bit of lip gloss onto the lid where you'll apply the orange, then apply the color over it.

4 **Eye shadow/highlight:** Use a small eye shadow brush to apply a pale shimmery green shadow from the center of the eyelids to under the brows.

5 **Eye liner/false eyelashes:** Line the base of the upper lashes with a bright blue liquid eye liner. Apply a set of very lightweight lashes.

6 **Lip color:** Define the lips with a bright orange matte lipstick.

simple creativity

Shirley Lord 70s

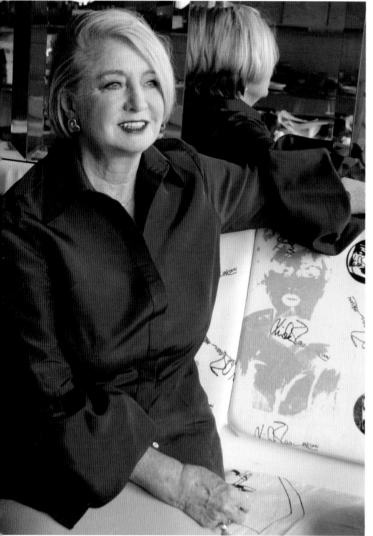

Shirley Lord, a former beauty director of *Vogue* and maven of the beauty industry, is a treasure trove of information. She's always been an inspiration to me and lives a full, active life as a journalist, author, and advisor to various companies. Shirley's late husband was A.M. Rosenthal, executive editor at the *New York Times*.

She believes in a simple makeup application for daytime, and strengthens her makeup look for the evening. She confided, "The tools and techniques are so advanced these days that 70 is the new 50. Brows are the most important: Make sure your brows and lashes are colored, since they often go white or gray before the hair does. If the brows disappear, then the whole structure of the face changes." It's mainly within the past few years that her skin has changed dramatically, and because she suffers from rosacea, her skin care regime needed serious updating. As for makeup, she says, "The best investment, rather than a facelift, is to consult with a really good professional makeup artist, as the contours of the face change with time. Eye makeup especially has always been a mystery for women, even for those who are comfortable working with their face."

For Shirley's base, I blended a light shade of cream base over her face and a light shade of concealer around her eyes. For women like Shirley who have heavy lids, it's important not to lighten the protruding area but to apply a deeper shade of matte eye shadow over it to lift it, then to accentuate the area under the brow with a slightly lighter color.

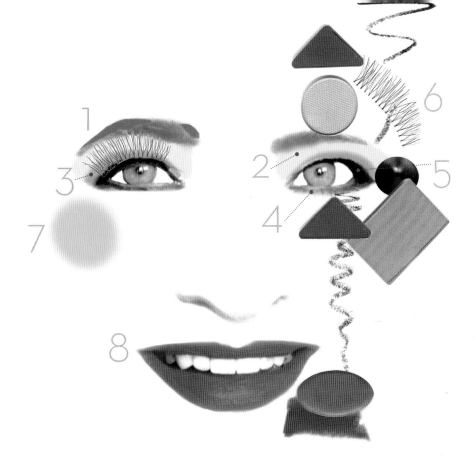

lunch at the carlyle

1 **Eyebrows:** Color and gently define lightly faded brows with a mixture of blond eyebrow pencil and a gold powder.

2 **Eye shadow/highlight:** With your large eye shadow brush, blend a matte apricot shadow over the brow.

3 **Eye shadow/midtone:** With your mini-eye shadow brush, apply a matte warm brown in the crease of the eye; blend it up into the apricot.

4 **Eye shadow/accent:** Using a mini-eye shadow brush, press bright blue eye shadow into the base of the lower lashes. If you would like the color to be stronger, use a pencil first.

5 **Eye liner/mascara:** To accentuate the eye, apply a black gel or cake eye liner at the base of the upper lashes. Apply black mascara to both the upper and lower lashes.

6 **False eyelashes:** These feathery brown eyelashes on a light base are a quick way to strengthen and enhance real lashes. They're softer-looking than thicker lashes on a dark base, so they're easy to wear during the day.

7 **Blush:** Dust a coral powder blush onto the cheekbones, blending it downward, to the apples of the cheeks. (If rosacea is a problem, don't apply blush to the apples of the cheeks; instead, just gently blend it to their tops.

8 **Lip color:** Define the lips with a coral pencil and apply a strong coral red lipstick with a lip brush to make sure the lips are well defined.

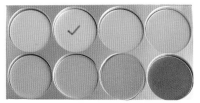

The color of cream base I used on Shirley.

smoky shimmer
Veronica Webb 40s

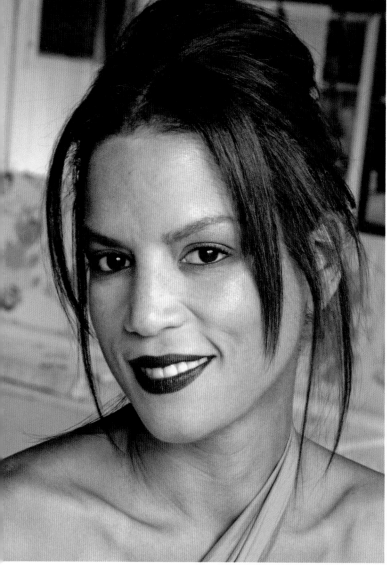

Veronica lives near my store in SoHo, and whenever I bump into her I see that she's becoming ever more beautiful as she matures. A busy mother, model, journalist, and spokesperson for the travel website Voyage.tv, she still manages to give fitness and grooming a high priority. She recently ran her first marathon, which may be one of the reasons her skin is so incredible.

The look I designed for Veronica features a smoky eye, but I departed from the traditional brown and black version with deep, rich matte burgundy and olive green. To keep this combination dark and smoky, I used an iridescent burgundy under the brows and over the edges of the olive. The step-by-step instructions for creating this eye are shown on pages 64–65; the variation shown here is even more colorful, with a touch of glitter-flecked violet shadow added to the very base of the upper lashes. To increase smokiness, use a mini–eye shadow brush to strengthen the crease with a heavy reapplication of olive, then blend it out into the iridescent burgundy highlight with the small shadow brush. Another option would be to apply black pencil at the base of both the upper and lower lashes, then to blend a black powder shadow over the pencil.

For Veronica's foundation, I used a damp sponge to apply a light gold liquid base to the entire face, then applied a medium yellow-toned cream base as a concealer, using a base brush to cover darker areas on the chin and redder areas around the nostrils, as well as to blend a little over the lids and under the eyes.

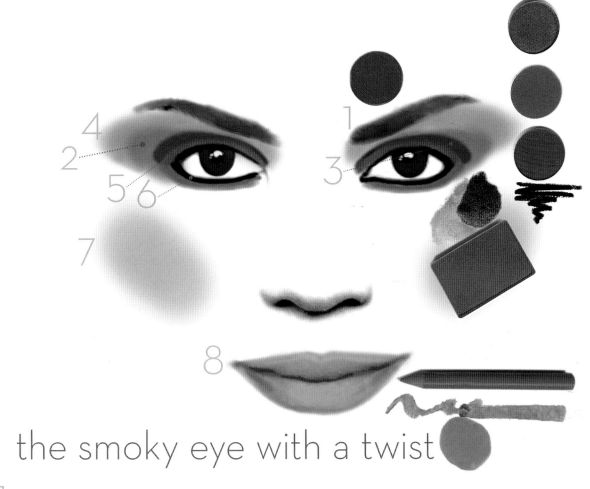

the smoky eye with a twist

1. **Eyebrows:** Fill in any sparse areas with brown powder.

2. **Eye shadow/midtone:** Use a mini–eye shadow brush to blend matte burgundy shadow around the entire eye. Apply it heavily at the very base of the lashes, then blend it into the crease. Blend and soften the shadow to extend it about one-eighth of an inch below the eye.

3. **Eye shadow/deep tone:** Blend a deep matte olive green into the crease with a small eye shadow brush, tapering it toward the ends of the brows.

4. **Eye shadow/highlight:** Blend an iridescent burgundy onto the brow bone and under the brow, from the inner corner past the outer corner, while softening the edge of the olive shadow.

5. **Eye shadow/accent:** Apply a violet shadow with flecks of glitter to the very base of the upper lashes.

6. **Eye liner/mascara:** Apply a soft black pencil to the inner rim of the lower lashes. Apply black mascara.

7. **Blush/powder:** Apply a matte berry blush to the underside of the cheekbone, then use a blusher brush to blend a soft iridescent mineral face powder along the top the cheekbone.

8. **Lip color:** Apply a brick lipstick (shown opposite), or an iridescent soft pink lipstick (shown above and on page 64). For the latter: Define the lips with a deeper pink pencil, soften the line by blending it into the lipstick, then add a touch of nude lip gel.

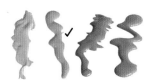

The color of liquid base I used on Veronica.

accentuating
personality

Nancy DeWeir Geaney 40s

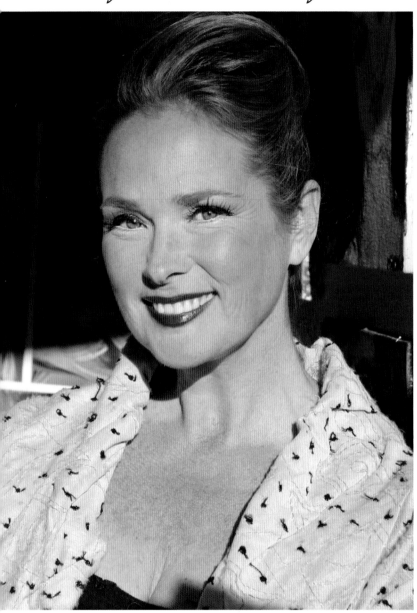

Nancy is a quilt artist and entrepreneur (darkhorsefarmdesigns. blogspot.com). We worked together many times while she was a top beauty model in the 1980s. Her fine skin and classic beauty still exude that same rare glow that made her such a success.

Her skin is redder now. The redness isn't unattractive, but because I planned to use bright colors on her eyes, it was essential that I first conceal her natural redness with a base so the colors wouldn't clash with her skin tone. I used a light beige liquid base, then applied a very light cream concealer under her eyes and to her eyelids before finishing her skin with a light dusting of translucent powder. The unusual combination of red and blue eye makeup with a dark lip color expresses Nancy's creative and positive personality.

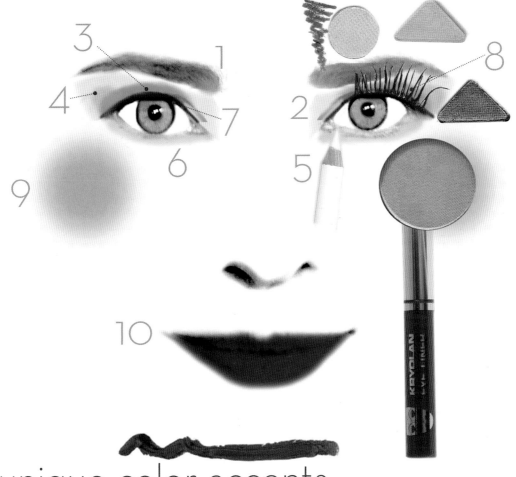

unique color accents

1 **Eyebrows:** Lightly accentuate the brows as needed; a blond eyebrow pencil was used here.

2 **Eye shadow/highlight:** Blend over the entire eyelid area in a pale matte pink-tinted ivory shadow using the large eye shadow brush.

3 **Eye shadow/midtone:** With the small eye shadow brush, blend stronger pink into the center of the eye, just above the crease.

4 **Eye shadow/accent:** Press into the eyelid a yellow-sand shade with your mini-eye shadow brush, just above the crease in the outer part of the eye.

5 **Eye pencil/white:** Apply a white pencil line to the inner rims and at the base of the lower lashes.

6 **Eye pencil/turquoise:** Apply a turquoise blue eye pencil line at the base of the lower lashes and blend it with the mini-eye shadow brush.

7 **Eye liner/mascara:** Apply a thin line of red liquid liner to the base of the upper lashes. Apply mascara to the upper lashes.

8 **False eyelashes:** Paint false eyelashes with red eye liner, let dry, then apply them.

9 **Blush:** Apply a little pink blush to the cheekbone.

10 **Lip color:** Apply a matte burgundy lipstick with a lip brush.

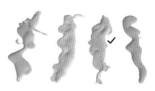

The color of liquid base I chose for Nancy.

studio 54 revisited
Coco Mitchell 50s

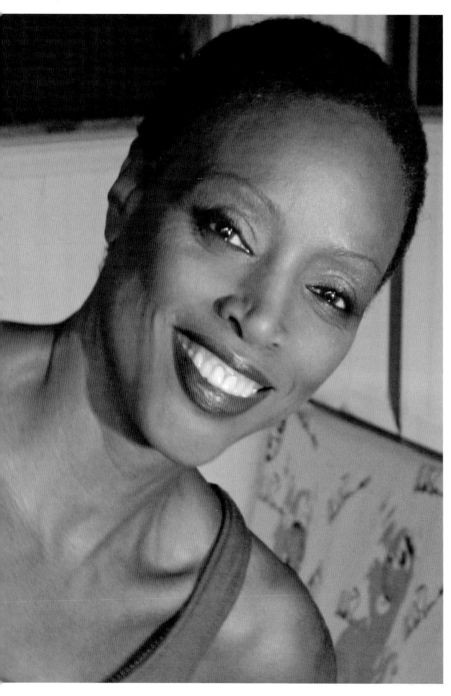

Coco was a teacher before she began pursuing a modeling career, which continues to take her all over the world. She also casts fashion shows and collaborates with fashion designers. She didn't wear makeup before modeling, but now she loves it and stays on top of the trends.

Coco's face and lids are wrinkle-free, so she can easily wear shimmery makeup on her lids. She has a great facial shape and features, so there are few complications when positioning the makeup application.

Coco's brows are very sparse and they suit her well in this way. I just gently defined them by making small strokes with a brunette pencil.

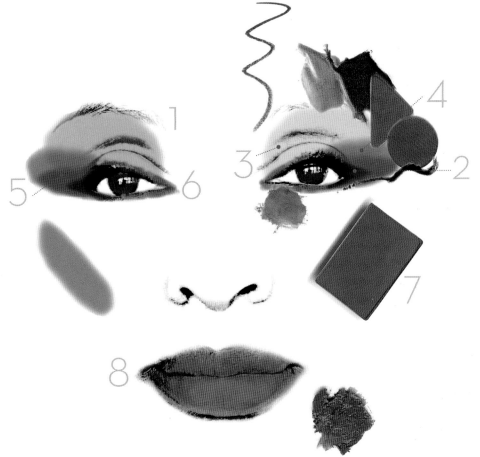

updated disco shimmer

1 **Eyebrows:** Shape and fill in brows with a brunette pencil as needed.

2 **Eye liner:** Apply black pencil inside the lower rims, then at the base of the upper and lower lashes. Use a mini-eye shadow brush to extend the line outward.

3 **Eye shadow/highlight:** Apply light pink iridescent shadow to the entire lid, then intensify it with a red iridescent shadow.

4 **Eye shadow/midtone:** Starting at the penciled area, blend matte fuchsia over the lighter colors, toward the ends of the brows.

5 **Eye shadow/deep tone:** Use a mini-eye shadow brush to press matte purple into the base of the lashes. Blend it over the penciling, lengthening the eye shape.

6 **Eye shadow/accent/mascara:** In the inner corners of the eyes, press a little iridescent lilac shadow on top of the matte violet and blend it outward. Finish the eyes with black mascara.

7 **Blush:** Apply deep russet cream blush slightly under the cheekbone, then blend it over the bone on a diagonal. Brush russet powder blush down the cheekbone and onto the apples of the cheeks.

8 **Lip color:** Apply a vibrant pink.

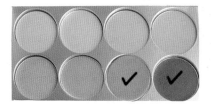

The colors of cream base that I chose for Coco.

BEAUTY CHALLENGE: evening out skin tone

To even out Coco's skin tone, I used a warm golden liquid base over her entire face, then added two cream bases, blending a little of the darker base onto the lighter patches and the lighter one onto the darker areas, finishing with a warm shade of powder.

wear color you love

Phyllis Molle 70s

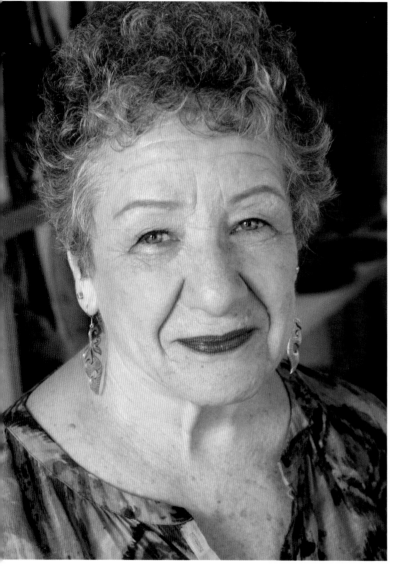

Phyllis is a retired nurse practitioner and a very strong personality. She likes vibrant color and looks great it in it. The day she came to my studio, she had on beautiful colorful glasses in bright blue and purple and a vivid turquoise top. Because she's vivacious and because, as a New Yorker, she often wears black, bright makeup is an appropriate accessory for her.

"I always wondered when one becomes 'sophisticated,'" Phyllis mused. "First I thought it was at 18 or 21 (before I was either), or maybe even 30. As I got older, I realized being sophisticated was related to how one learned to be comfortable in the world and how one might help others do the same. It has nothing to do with age. Makeup makes my face come alive. I don't wear a lot of makeup daily, but it's nice to learn what to do for special occasions. It offers a whole sense of *joie de vivre*." Her daily makeup routine includes mascara and a lipstick called "Love That Pink" by Revlon, which she's been wearing for many years.

For Phyllis's base, I applied a cream base in a medium beige shade, then a medium light concealer to the lids and under the eyes, taking care to avoid emphasizing the lines there. For the first makeup look, we decided to do a soft blue eye. Phyllis has small eyes, so we made sure to not cover the entire lid with color, which would have overpowered them. We also didn't apply color under the eyes, again to avoid drawing attention to the lines.

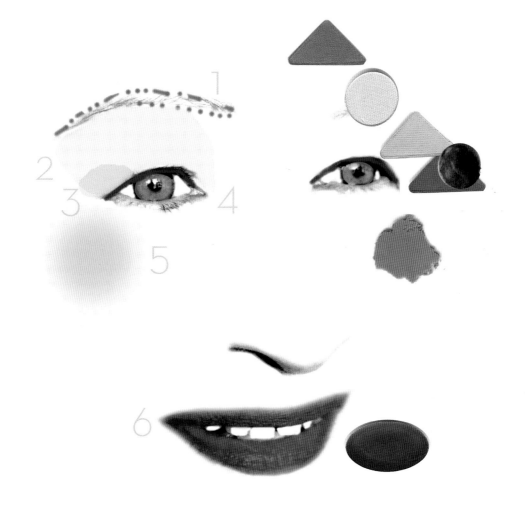

everyday brights

1. **Eyebrows:** Shape and color the eyebrows as needed. Here a gray powder shadow was lightly applied with an angled brow brush.

2. **Eye shadow/highlight:** Blend a pale matte cream color under the eyebrows on the brow bone using a large eye shadow brush.

3. **Eye shadow/accent:** With the mini-eye shadow brush, blend a bright turquoise with a touch of blue added from the base of the lashes past the crease. Take care not to go past the crease too far on the inside of the eye and to blend the color into the cream shade so as not to be obvious.

4. **Eye liner/mascara:** Accent the eyes using the eye liner brush and a dark blue gel liner. Finish the eyes with black mascara.

5. **Blush/powder:** Blend in a little pink cream blush over the cheekbone. (At this point, I applied a very light dusting of translucent powder to the cheeks and chin and around the nose—the areas that look better when they're matte.)

6. **Lip color:** Apply a soft blue-red (in this case, red currant).

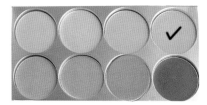

The color of cream base I chose for Phyllis.

evening color

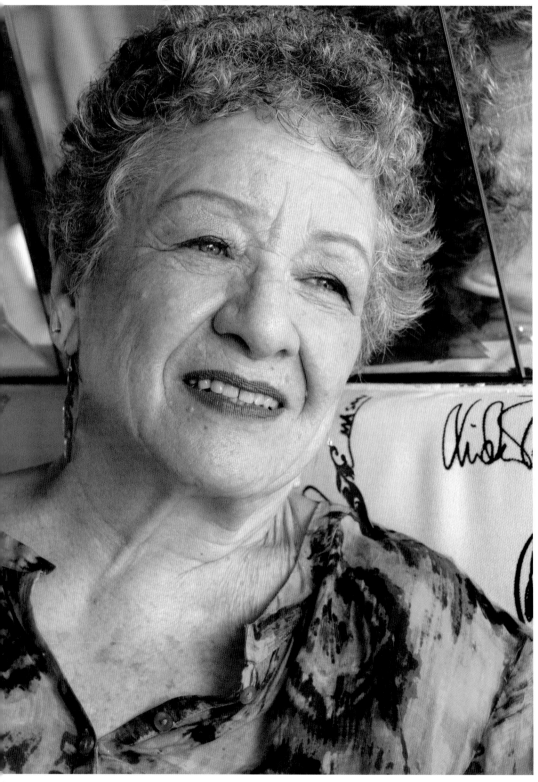

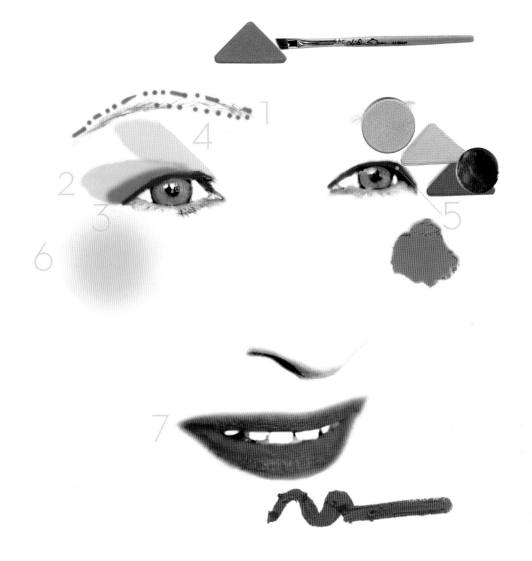

1 **Eyebrows:** Shape and color the eyebrows as needed; here I lightly applied a gray powder shadow with an angled brow brush.

2 **Eye shadow/midtone:** With the mini-eye shadow brush, blend an ample amount of turquoise past the crease, working outward and upward.

3 **Eye shadow/accent:** Press blue eye shadow into the base of the lashes in the outer part of the eye. Blend it into the turquoise to strengthen it, but don't take it as far as the turquoise.

4 **Eye shadow/highlight:** Blend in beige with a fleck of iridescence across the eyelid on a diagonal. This should go over the edge of the color beneath to soften it.

5 **Eye liner/mascara:** Apply dark blue gel liner using an eye liner brush. Finish the eyes with black mascara.

6 **Blush/powder:** Blend in a little pink cream blush over the cheekbone. (At this point, I applied very little powder, only to the cheeks and chin and around the nose.)

7 **Lip color:** Apply a vibrant blue-pink.

creating a mood
with color

Frederique van der Wal 40s

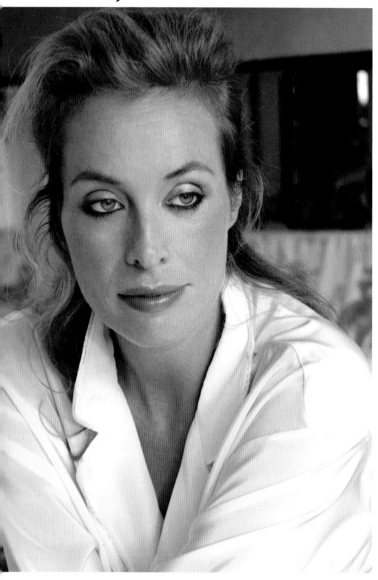

Frederique has had a very successful career as a model, working for Victoria's Secret and *Sports Illustrated* among other high-profile clients, and she remains in high demand for photo shoots and acting work. The Dutch native is also the owner of Frederique's Choice (FrederiquesChoice.com), an online floral and gift company she founded in 2005 after the Dutch government named a pink lily in her honor.

For her beauty routine, Frederique uses moisturizer and sunscreen religiously and makes sure to wash her face every night. While growing up in Holland, she developed a healthy appreciation for food but never diets, and keeps fit by doing yoga, tennis, Pilates, and riding her bike as much as possible.

Though Frederique never wears base when she does her own makeup, she isn't intimidated by it because of the makeup artists she's worked with as a model, so I used a beige cream base with a yellow undertone and a light dusting of translucent powder. I was inspired to accentuate her signature "bedroom eyes" with a light shimmery gold on her lids, hints of bright yellow-orange and turquoise (if your eyes are like Frederique's and aren't sunken in the inner corners, you can get away with a touch of bright color there) and brown pencil lining her lower lashes. To keep the emphasis on the eyes, I was careful to not use anything too strong on her cheekbones and lips.

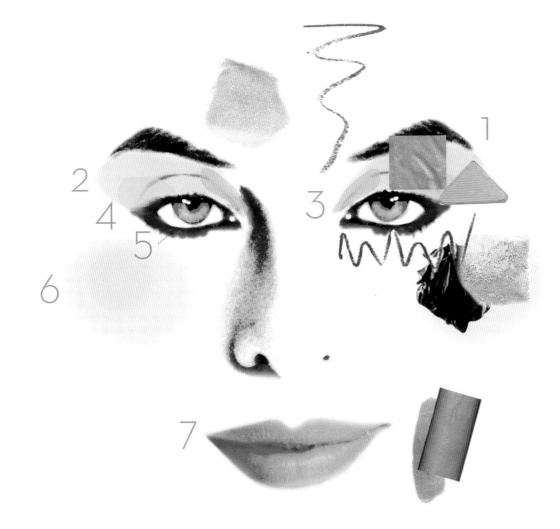

playing up seductive eyes

1 **Eyebrows:** Define brows with a blond pencil.

2 **Eye shadow/highlight:** Dust a loose yellow-gold shadow all over the lid.

3 **Eye shadow/accent:** For this look I used a pop of a loose powder eyeshadow in yellow-orange in the inner corner of the eyes.

4 **Eye shadow/midtone:** Apply aqua to the outer third of the lid, angling it up toward the end of the brow to create a visual lift.

5 **Eye liner:** With a brown eye pencil, line the inner and outer rims of the lower lashes, then soften and extend the shading slightly beyond the outer corners with the mini-eye shadow brush.

6 **Blush:** Blend a minute amount of reddish brown cream blush (good for every day) onto cheekbones. Add a slight dusting of pink mineral blush over the cheekbone, blending it down lightly onto the cheeks.

7 **Lip color:** Apply a light-colored lip gloss, then dab nude lipstick in the center of the lips.

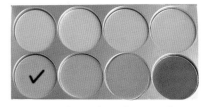

The color of cream base I chose for Frederique.

warm and cool palettes

Jan Jaffe 60's

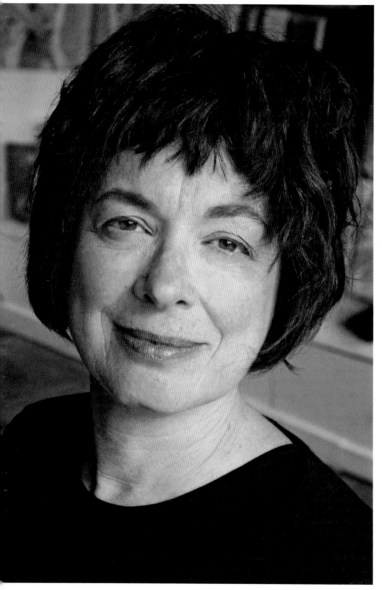

Jan has been a client of mine for 10 years. When she first came to see me she was 50 and wore little makeup. She wasn't interested in a natural look but also didn't want one that was caked on, heavy, or complicated. Her good skin and great features made her an easy candidate for unique color combinations, so I introduced her to colored eye shadows and bright lipsticks.

For her first look, my approach was to lift her eyes with a soft color on the lids and a touch of either a brighter or darker color over it, in the outer corners, always using mattes or semi-mattes that would blend easily into her skin. I chose not to use any base on her skin, but just a pale cream concealer. Jan doesn't normally wear eye liner, but I added a little green gel liner at the base of the upper lashes in the outer third of her eye. She also doesn't usually wear blush, but I applied a red powder in a color that matches her natural redness to her cheekbones, starting high and blending lightly downward onto the apples of the cheeks. I completed the look with a black lip gloss to slightly deepen the color of her lips.

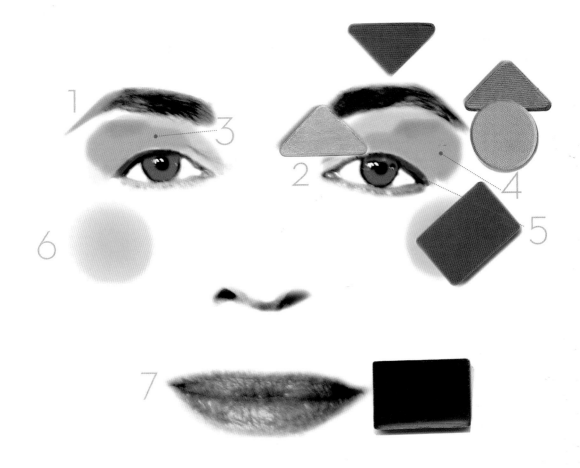

a cool, soft palette

1 **Eyebrows:** Fill in and adjust the brows as needed. For Jan I applied a burgundy eye shadow with an angled brow brush to soften the difference between her brow and hair color and to strengthen the line of her right brow.

2 **Eye shadow/highlight:** Use a small eye shadow brush to blend light blue eye shadow from the inner corners of the eyes to the brows.

3 **Eye shadow/midtone:** Blend a lime-green shadow from the center of the lids to the brows with a small eye shadow brush.

4 **Eye shadow/accent:** Blend a soft semipearl beige eye shadow from the base of the lashes in the outer corners upward and outward.

5 **Eye liner/mascara:** Apply a thin line of green gel eye liner to the base of the upper lashes. Finish the eyes with black mascara.

6 **Blush:** Blend a touch of a matte red powder blush on the cheekbones.

7 **Lip color:** Deepen the natural color of the lips with black lip gloss.

a warm, bright palette

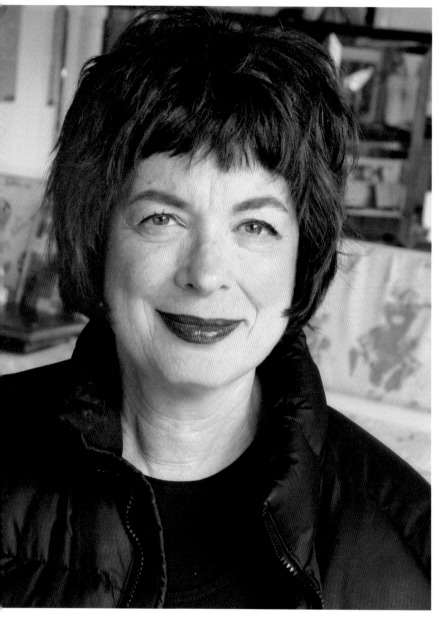

Jan wanted another look, and asked about yellow and orange for her eyes. I designed one that brightened her face dramatically by blending yellow shadow from the base of the lashes upward and outward and pressing orange over the yellow in the outer upper corners of the eyes, then blending it upward past the crease. I intensified the eyes with red eye liner and black mascara. I also encouraged her to try a ruby red lipstick; with her fuller lips, it was better to forgo pencil liner, which would have made them too heavy and defined. For this look we used base, concealer, and powder.

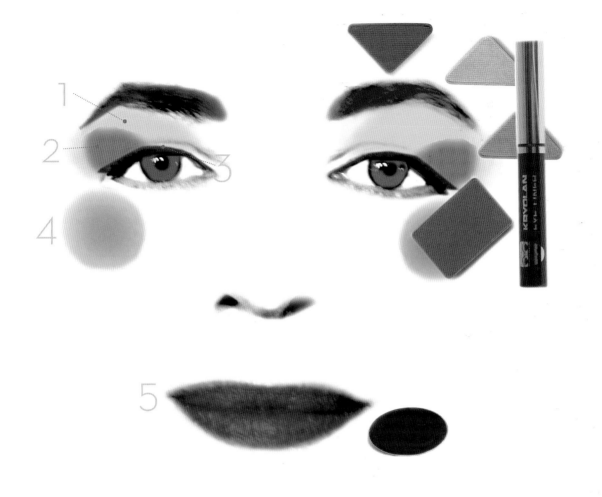

1 **Eye shadow/highlight:** Blend soft yellow eye shadow from the base
of the lashes upward toward the brows.

2 **Eye shadow/deep tone:** Press in bright orange at the base of the upper
lashes in the outer corners and blend it past the crease of the eye.

3 **Eye liner/mascara:** Apply a thin line of red liner to the base of the upper lashes.
Finish the eyes with black mascara.

4 **Blush:** Blend a touch of matte red powder blush on the cheekbones.

5 **Lip color:** Define the lips with ruby red lipstick.

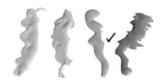

The color of liquid base
I choose for Jan.

resources

A list of publications and sites geared toward women who are looking for information, advice, and inspiration on makeup and skincare, fashion, style, and health.

Beauty

Glamour
Glamour.com
Offers features on fashion, beauty, and a contemporary lifestyle.

More
More.com
Celebrates women over 40, with articles on beauty, health, fashion, and more.

Stylelist.com
Reports on the latest beauty products and fashion trends.
Totalbeauty.com
Features beauty product reviews, beauty advice, and how-to videos.

Vogue
Vogue.com
Authoritative news and features on fashion, beauty, collections, and culture.

Health and wellness
Whole Living
WholeLiving.com
Tips for healthy eating, fitness, and mental well-being.

Women.WebMD.com
Comprehensive information on healthy living and well-being.

Shopping
Skinstore.com
Carries a large array of brand-name products for all skincare needs. Features an education center with information on specific topics.

index

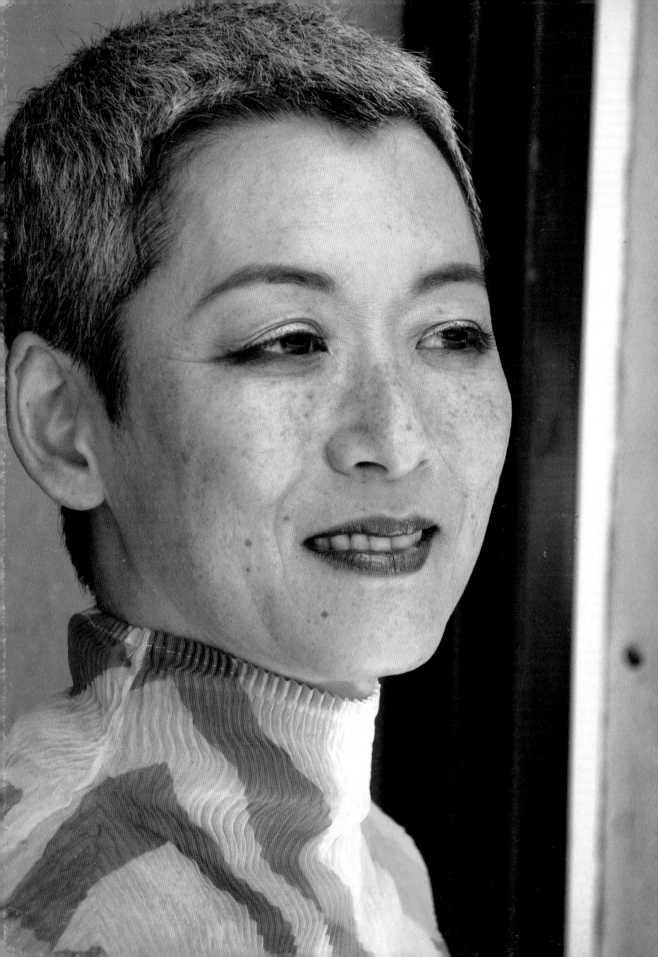